The Arthritis Foundation's Guide to
GOOD LIVING
With
Fibromyalgia

The Arthritis Foundation's Guide to
GOOD LIVING
With
Fibromyalgia

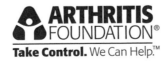

An Official Publication
of the Arthritis Foundation

Published by
Arthritis Foundation
1330 West Peachtree Street
Atlanta, GA 30309

Printed in the United States of America
1st Printing 2001

Library of Congress Card Catalog Number: 00-111406

ISBN: 0-912423-26-9

Table of Contents

PART ONE: LEARN ALL YOU CAN

Foreword

Fibromyalgia is a common condition affecting 3.7 million Americans. Fibromyalgia causes scattered pain, lack of energy, poor sleep and myriad other signs and symptoms. Because symptoms of many diseases cause similar complaints, diagnosis is difficult. Often many weeks or months go by before the person with fibromyalgia or the doctor recognizes what is wrong. During this time the results of an examination by the doctor are normal, as are routine studies like blood tests, urinalysis and X-rays. But reassurances that nothing is wrong provide little relief, and patient and doctor become equally frustrated that the symptoms refuse to go away. Both may worry that a serious illness remains unrevealed, adding to the patient's anxiety.

In most people with fibromyalgia, symptoms improve once a diagnosis is made and a course of treatment begins. Indeed, doctors have much to recommend in terms of medicines or physical therapy that can help pain and other symptoms. However, the real key to successful treatment requires an active participation – a take-charge attitude – by the person with fibromyalgia. This active role includes learning about the condition, its causes and, in particular, what changes you can make in your daily life that help. This book – *The Arthritis Foundation's Guide to Good Living With Fibromyalgia* – is a great resource for learning about fibromyalgia and how a person with the condition can improve his or her life.

John H. Klippel, MD
Medical Director
Arthritis Foundation, Atlanta, GA

For more information about fibromyalgia, including how to enroll in specially designed exercise classes or in a Fibromyalgia Self-Help Course in your area, contact your local Arthritis Foundation chapter by calling 800-283-7800, or log on to www.arthritis.org on the Internet.

Acknowledgments

The Arthritis Foundation's Guide to Good Living With Fibromyalgia is written for people who have fibromyalgia, and for their families and friends. While this book should not take the place of the advice and treatment that your physicians and other healthcare professionals provide, it may help you better understand your fibromyalgia. Through this deeper knowledge, you can take a more active role in self-managing your condition.

This book is inspired by the Arthritis Foundation's Fibromyalgia Self-Help Course, a program of self-management developed in the late 1980s and originally supported by the Norma Borie Fibromyalgia Research and Education Program Fund, and by the Chronic Disease Self-Management Course, developed by Kate Lorig, RN, DrPH, and her colleagues at the Stanford Arthritis Center.

This book was reviewed for medical accuracy by John H. Klippel, MD, Medical Director of the Arthritis Foundation; Laurence Bradley, PhD, of the University of Alabama, Birmingham; Daniel J. Clauw, MD, of Georgetown University Hospital in Washington, DC; Don L. Goldenberg, MD, of Newton-Wellesley Hospital in Newton, MA; and Patricia Grosklaus, PT, of Atlanta, GA. The development of the book also included reviews and suggestions by Arthritis Foundation volunteers and staff around the country.

Special thanks go to Dorothy Foltz-Gray, who wrote the text. The editorial director of the book is Susan Bernstein. The art director of the book is Susan Siracusa.

Introduction

The most important person managing your fibromyalgia is *you*. That's why the Arthritis Foundation organized this book around the five most significant habits you can develop to manage your condition. We're convinced that if you follow the advice the book offers, you can deal with your fibromyalgia more effectively.

The first step for anyone in managing a medical problem is to learn as much as possible about his or her condition. The more you know about the physical and mental landscape of fibromyalgia, its causes and treatments, the better equipped you will be to handle the changes fibromyalgia brings to your life. Now more than ever before, medical research is yielding new information about both conventional and alternative therapies for treating the condition's many symptoms.

As important as your education is the relationship you form with the doctors, nurses and specialists who will work with you to manage your condition. Doctors vary as much as patients do, and finding one whom you feel confident about and comfortable with will affect the quality of your care. Understanding what your doctor needs and expects from you also will affect your treatment, psychologically and physically.

No matter what your doctor recommends, you're the only person who can implement the therapies you decide on together. There is no quick fix for fibromyalgia. Your surest route to feeling better depends on the daily habits you develop. Research has proven that a healthy diet, regular exercise and satisfying personal relationships are all essential features of well-being. None of those things, together or separately, can make fibromyalgia disappear, but each is an important part of staying and feeling well.

Although you will have days when you feel that fibromyalgia is the boss, you can control many of the choices that will affect how you feel. Learning to set goals, solve problems and prioritize how you spend your energy will help you deal with this condition. The same is true for managing pain, fatigue and sleep. The more you learn about ways to alter the aspects of your life that work against your fibromyalgia, the better you will feel.

Depression, grief and stress can all accompany fibromyalgia. Accepting, understanding and working through those tough emotions is an important habit, as crucial as daily exercise or self-education. This book will begin to show you how to deal with fibromyalgia's many challenges.

Unfortunately, fibromyalgia can't be cured by pills or surgery. With education, hard work and persistence, you can achieve good living with this condition. With a commitment to help yourself, you *can* feel better. That option lies within your power. Consider this book a resource and guide in the journey to a better life.

Part One

Learn All You Can

Chapter 1

Understanding Fibromyalgia:

A Mysterious, Chronic Condition

Your first hint of fibromyalgia may be aching, painful muscles, fatigue and disturbed sleep. Your shoulders hurt, and come to think of it, so do your knees and hips. Your sleep is troubled, and you can't remember the last time you woke refreshed. You may have headaches and stomach pain, and just walking to the mailbox feels like more exercise that you can or want to manage. In many places on your body, even a little pressure feels painful. You take aspirin and you rest, but nothing seems to help much. Mostly, you feel miserable and bewildered: "What on earth is happening to my body?" you may ask yourself. Your physician may not be able to diagnose the cause of these symptoms at first, subjecting you to many tests that do not confirm the source of your problems.

What Is Fibromyalgia?

You may be confused about your symptoms, and frustrated by the difficulty in finding a diagnosis, but you're in good company. Now classified as one of 150 conditions related to arthritis, fibromyalgia affects as many as 3.7 million Americans. Fibromyalgia affects more women than men.

Fibromyalgia long bewildered the medical profession. (See sidebar, p. 5.) For many years, fibromyalgia was believed to be myth, a story in an aching woman's head, a figment of troubled minds. Until 1990, the condition lacked both a name and criteria for diagnosis. That year, the American College of Rheumatology (ACR), an association of 5,000 *rheumatologists* (doctors who specialize in treating diseases of the musculoskeletal system) in the United States and Canada, released its criteria for diagnosing fibromyalgia. Having fibromyalgia means you have all of the following symptoms:

• A history of widespread pain on both sides of the body, above and below the waist, present for at least three months;

• Pain in at least 11 of 18 tender point sites, and in all four quadrants of the body if the length and width of the body were each divided in half.

Tender points are areas of the body that are particularly sensitive to pressure. Although fibromyalgia is diagnosed by finding pain in these specific points, people with fibromyalgia may experience pain and tenderness virtually anywhere in their body. Tender points merely represent some of the most common areas of pain (see diagram at right). The location of some of these tender points is similar to other common muscle disorders, such as lateral epicondylitis or *tennis elbow* (painful inflammation of the elbow tendons), and *trochanteric bursitis* (irritation of certain muscle attachments outside the hip). Each tender point almost always matches a "mirror" point in the same place on the opposite side of the body. Sometimes people won't notice the tender sites until a rheumatologist or other trained specialist applies pressure. Not all physicians know how to evaluate tender points.

Unlike *arthritis*, a disease that involves joint inflammation, fibromyalgia does not damage joints or cause inflammation. Because its symptoms occur in muscles and joints, doctors classify it as *soft-tissue rheumatism*, a broad term including a group of disorders that cause pain and stiffness around the joints and in muscles and bones. According to Daniel J. Wallace, MD, author of the 1999 book *Making Sense of Fibromyalgia* (Oxford University Press), people who are diagnosed

early and self-manage their symptoms tend to improve. Self-management of fibromyalgia may include having a nutritious diet, cutting back on alcohol, quitting smoking, getting proper exercise, finding techniques for reducing stress and learning to work cooperatively with doctors and other health-care professionals to find medications or other ways to alleviate symptoms.

Common Symptoms in Adults

No two people experience exactly the same fibromyalgia symptoms to exactly the same degree, and the symptoms in children differ somewhat from those of adults (see "Children and Fibromyalgia," page 8).

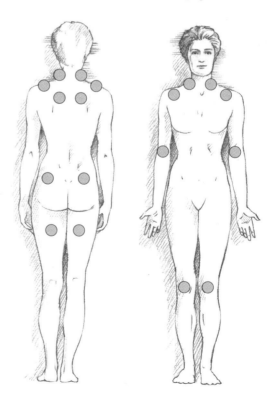

JOINTS USUALLY AFFECTED BY FIBROMYALGIA

Personally Speaking   Stories from real people with fibromyalgia

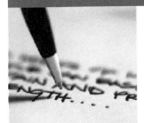

"People always told me I looked older than my age. I looked 20 when I was 12. At 28, I felt 100 years old. I was tired, not "take-a-nap" tired or "up-late-the-night-before" tired, but an aching tired that was deep in my bones.

"I received advice from every caring, well-intentioned person in my life. 'Eat less carbohydrates, sleep more, sleep less, cut out all sugar, take hot baths, take cold showers, _exercise_.' How do you smile and say 'thank you,' when the only thing you want is for someone to understand that even the mere thought of exercise, of bending and stretching, caused the aches to intensify? The idea of doing any of these things was exhausting.

A Name for the Pain
Julie Schneider,
Atlanta, GA

"I searched the Internet for answers to the shooting pains, the aches, the exhaustion. It always came up as 'depression.' I would plug in every symptom again and again. I found remedies to each individual symptom, but nothing that tied it all together. I didn't want to be depressed. I didn't want to have a list of symptoms. I wanted to have something with a name or nothing at all.

"Four months after my 29th birthday, two years after I began having these symptoms, I went to a new doctor. I had had an unbearable week of pain in my lower back. It was a new spot, a new pain and the end to my ignoring-it-all-away attitude. All I was looking for was validation, someone to make my pain real. I told my doctor everything, every crazy thought, every scary symptom and every frustrating moment.

"I had a battery of blood tests for everything from lupus to rheumatoid arthritis. All the tests came back negative. I was thankful and disheartened in the same moment. After a few more consultations and an appointment with a rheumatologist, I was diagnosed with fibromyalgia.

"I learned that I was actually sleeping too much but not achieving deep sleep. Now I take a medication that helps me reach that level of serenity every night. I actually sleep, a healthy, fulfilling, restful sleep.

"Sometimes I wake up with moments of stiffness. I have exercises and stretches to ease the stiffness. Now, I'm motivated to do them. After the first few days of stretching, it got easier and it actually began to make me feel better.

"Sometimes I have quick, shooting pains in my back, arms and legs. I know I need to stop and close my eyes, not fight the pain or get scared. It will pass. I know that now. I know so much now that I didn't know before. I know that I am in control of this disease. I know that I must take responsibility for my health. I know that I am thankful it is not terminal or even imaginary. Most of all I know that I am not alone and that I can not only cope, but I can overcome."

However, many people with fibromyalgia experience common symptoms and many of these symptoms, are interrelated. For example, fibromyalgia pain can disturb sleep and heighten fatigue. Poor sleep and increased fatigue may lead to limiting one's activities, which may dampen spirits and lead to depression. Depression at the same time often disturbs sleep.

PAIN

Muscle pain is the most prominent and common symptom of fibromyalgia. Although it is generally felt all over, this pain may start in one region, such as the neck and shoulders, and spread to other regions. Pain may be intense in one area, then disappear, only to appear in another area. Although pain may occur around the joints, the joints themselves are not affected as they are in inflammatory forms of arthritis.

Some people with fibromyalgia describe the pain as knife-like in intensity; others compare it to an all-over muscle cramp. For some, the pain is severe. It can vary depending on time, weather, sleep patterns, the point in a woman's menstrual cycle, activity and stress levels. Most people with fibromyalgia say that some pain is always present, and many say it feels like a persistent flu.

FATIGUE

Between 60 percent and 80 percent of people with fibromyalgia report moderate to severe fatigue. Many often wake up feeling tired, even after sleeping through the night. Although sleeplessness contributes to fatigue,

so can other factors, such as stress, depression, illness, poor diet, overwork and medication.

Fatigue also has many forms. It can mean listlessness, decreased exercise endurance, mental or physical exhaustion, or sleepiness that varies during the day and from one day to the next.

About 50 percent to 70 percent of fibromyalgia patients may also have *chronic fatigue syndrome*, a flu-like illness accompanied not only by fatigue but also by a sore throat, painful glands and a sensation of fever.

SLEEP DISTURBANCE

Scientific studies demonstrate that between 60 percent and 90 percent of people with fibromyalgia have abnormal sleep patterns. They may find it hard to fall asleep, and/or they may wake up frequently once they do. In fact, sleep problems may be one cause of the condition. During normal deep sleep (called *delta* sleep) the body produces a growth hormone that repairs and restores muscle. Fibromyalgia patients get little deep sleep. This problem may also explain why many people with the condition produce less growth hormone than people who get enough deep sleep. Scientists speculate that lower than normal levels of growth hormone may leave muscles more vulnerable to trauma. See Chapter 12 for more information on sleep.

DEPRESSION AND ANXIETY

Mood changes are common in fibromyalgia. Many people with the condition report feeling "blue" or "down," although only approximately 25 percent are considered clinically depressed, a condition requiring the care of a mental-health professional such as a *psychiatrist* (see Chapter 14). Some people also feel anxious. Some researchers feel there may be a biological link between fibromyalgia and some forms of depression and chronic anxiety, but this possible link is still unclear.

COGNITIVE DIFFICULTIES

Many people with fibromyalgia may experience *cognitive disturbance*, popularly known as *fibro fog*. They may experience feelings of confusion, lapses in memory, word mix-ups and difficulty concentrating. These problems also are common in sleep-deprived people. In fact, one 1997 study published in the *Journal of Rheumatology* suggests that the *cognitive*, or mental, difficulties in those with fibromyalgia may be a result of poor sleep. In the study,

10 women with fibromyalgia and a control group of nine women without the condition were asked to complete a set of cognitive tasks. Those with fibromyalgia performed complex memory tasks more slowly than the control group although with the same accuracy. Also brain scan studies performed by researchers at the University of Alabama have shown that from time to time, people with fibromyalgia do not receive enough oxygen in different parts of their brain. One possible reason is that part of their nervous systems, the *autonomic nervous system,* is off-kilter, causing changes in the brain's blood vessels.

OTHER SIGNS AND SYMPTOMS

Many physical problems may accompany fibromyalgia, causing additional pain, discomfort and frustration. You may get headaches, for example, especially muscular or tension

Fibromyalgia's Past:

Medical literature began discussing the symptoms of fibromyalgia in the early 1900s, but recognition and treatment of the condition did not accelerate until the early 1980s. By 1989, the respected *Textbook on Rheumatology, 3rd edition* included a chapter on fibrositis, a term for the little-understood condition at that time. But the chapter's author, Robert M. Bennett, MD, professor of medicine and director of the division of arthritis and rheumatic diseases at Oregon Health Sciences University in Portland, pointed out that the name didn't really fit. Fibrositis stems from Latin, meaning inflammation ("itis") of fibrous tissue ("fibro"). Fibromyalgia does not cause inflammation as arthritis does. A year later, the American College of Rheumatology (ACR) agreed that the condition should be called *fibromyalgia syndrome*. By adding the Greek words "mys" and "algia," meaning muscle pain, the term becomes a more accurate description of the syndrome, which is marked by widespread muscle pain and tenderness.

headaches and *migraines*. These headaches can be treated with a variety of drugs, including acetaminophen and nonsteroidal anti-inflammatory drugs (see Chapter 2) or a combination painkiller and muscle relaxant such as *Esgic* (butalbital with acetaminophen and caffeine). Preventive medications, such as calcium-channel blockers, tricyclic antidepressants and beta blockers also can be helpful. In some cases, massage or relaxation techniques are effective.

People with fibromyalgia also may experience bladder irritability and spasms resulting in a frequent urge to urinate, as well as *irritable bowel syndrome*, a condition marked by alternating constipation and diarrhea. The skin may temporarily change color because of sensitivity to temperature and moisture. Hands, arms, feet, legs or face may tingle or become numb. Problems with the jaw, such as *temporomandibular joint disorder* (TMJ), pre-menstrual discomfort, painful menstruation, dizziness and abdominal pain also can occur.

About 10 percent of people with fibromyalgia also have *restless leg syndrome*, which causes their legs to jump with spasms during sleep. These symptoms can come and go, and they may become worse during times of illness, stress or excessive physical exertion.

WHO GETS FIBROMYALGIA?

Fibromyalgia affects one out of every 50 Americans. Although the majority of those who have it are women between the ages of 40 and 75, it affects men, young women and children as well.

Men or women with other rheumatic diseases such as *rheumatoid arthritis* (a chronic, inflammatory autoimmune disease involving the joints that causes pain, swelling and deformity) and *lupus* (an inflammatory autoimmune disease of the connective tissue that can involve skin, joints, kidneys, blood and other organs) are at greater risk for fibromyalgia. For example, about 20 percent to 30 percent of those with rheumatoid arthritis also develop fibromyalgia, although no one knows the exact reason. There does not seem to be a cause-and-effect relationship between the two conditions; generally, when rheumatoid arthritis improves through treatment, fibromyalgia does not improve.

Fibromyalgia sometimes occurs in more than one member of the same family, but doctors have not verified a hereditary link or common genetic type. This prevalence within families could occur simply because fibromyalgia is a common condition. However several recent studies have found a possible link between genetic markers called *human leukocyte antigens*, or HLAs, and fibromyalgia. Although researchers are cautious about interpreting the findings, they suggest the possible existence of a gene that predisposes a person to develop fibromyalgia.

Children and Fibromyalgia

Although fibromyalgia is most common in adult women, the disorder has become increasingly prevalent in adolescents, further evidence of a possible connection between hormones and fibromyalgia. Of the 10,000 children in the United States diagnosed with

Personally Speaking

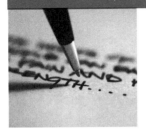

"Our daughter's doctor looked at us and said, 'Karen has fibromyalgia.' 'Fibro *what?*' we asked. The doctor gave my husband Ron and me a booklet on children and fibromyalgia that included a list of symptoms. What a relief to find out that many of our 14-year-old's complaints were linked to the condition and not individual ailments.

Raising a Child Who Has Fibromyalgia
Arlene Kaizer,
West Hartford, CT

"We joined a support group for children and their parents. Ron was too depressed to go back after the first meeting, but I continued to attend. The veteran parents gave me clues on how to deal with the school and on Karen's rights. They also told me about new medical theories and medicines. They gave me an application for a handicapped parking permit and offered a safe place to vent my frustration and anger.

Joining associations, going to conferences, reading books and articles has increased my knowledge, and I understand better what Karen is going through. Now I can suggest ways for her to manage. I know better ways to approach her school and to discuss different treatments with her doctors. I'm more informed as I do battle with the insurance company.

"I wish I could say dealing with a sick child is easier than at first. But it is just different. When Karen was diagnosed, we worried about every ache and pain she had. We panicked at her stomach pains, fearing they might be signs of appendicitis. Her hand tremors were spooky, but now we take them in stride. She still gets severe headaches, but we don't agonize that they might be symptoms of a tumor.

"The ways we manage as a family have evolved slowly and sometimes painfully. Still, it's tough figuring out if Karen's actions are normal teenage stuff or the result of fibromyalgia. For example, we feel homework and rest should come first. Karen doesn't. She feels best at night so that's when she wants to socialize. After many tearful arguments and shouting, Ron and I have become more lax in letting Karen go out at night. We've come to believe that her social life is necessary for her mental health and well-being. She's happier when she can see her friends. It's what 'normal' teenagers do.

"Fortunately, the administration at Karen's school has been wonderful about making accommodations for Karen. On the first day of each school year, Karen gives her teachers a packet of information including a brochure about fibromyalgia, a *Guidelines for Schools* booklet published by the National Chronic Fatigue and Immune Dysfunction Syndrome Foundation, a letter explaining her difficulties, and a request to call me if a problem comes up. I also keep the school nurse and Karen's guidance counselor updated on Karen's condition. They, in turn, are Karen's greatest advocates.

"Having a sense of humor helps us relieve tension and keeps us sane. We've learned to take things day by day. Each one is an adventure of new symptoms and new emotions."

the syndrome, 90 percent are adolescents. Of children with chronic pain syndromes, 25 percent to 40 percent fulfill the criteria for juvenile fibromyalgia syndrome.

Fibromyalgia in children first was reported in medical literature in 1985 by Muhammad B. Yunus, MD, of the University of Illinois College of Medicine. Many of the symptoms seen by Dr. Yunus and his colleagues were similar to those seen in adults with fibromyalgia, but the children had fewer tender points. Because the American College of Rheumatology has developed criteria for diagnosing adults only, doctors don't yet know if these criteria are valid for children also.

Still, up to 28 percent of adults with fibromyalgia report that their symptoms began during childhood. A study of 33 children with fibromyalgia, conducted by Dr. Yunus, identified the following symptoms:

- generalized aches and pains
- stiffness
- morning fatigue
- chronic headaches
- irritable bowel syndrome

According to the *Primer on the Rheumatic Diseases, 11th Ed.*, published by the Arthritis Foundation, children with fibromyalgia, like adults, often sleep poorly. The study by Dr. Yunus also notes that noisy surroundings, poor sleep, significant family dysfunction and depression are common among children with the syndrome.

For treating children with fibromyalgia, doctors have had some success with combinations of physical therapy, exercise, oral or injected glucocorticoids and psychological counseling. Despite the initial harshness of the condition, several studies suggest that with aggressive treatment there is a marked improvement in 80 percent of children and adolescents within one to three years of onset.

PARENTING A CHILD WITH FIBROMYALGIA

If your child has fibromyalgia, then family, friends, peers and especially school officials need to understand the various symptoms of the condition, such as pain, fatigue or cognitive disturbance. Talk with teachers and school staff about your child's condition, and discuss any difficulties he or she may have doing normal school activities such as sports. Encourage your child to remain active, get plenty of exercise and rest, and lead as normal a life as possible.

Many organizations can provide valuable information about fibromyalgia and how it affects children. To begin, contact the American Juvenile Arthritis Organization (AJAO), a council of the Arthritis Foundation, at 404/965-7538. They may be able to provide information or guidance on raising a child with fibromyalgia.

The Arthritis Foundation produces a variety of informative materials about fibromyalgia and the challenges children with rheumatic diseases and related conditions face. The Foundation publishes a book, *Raising a Child with Arthritis,* that offers useful guidance for the parents of children with fibromyalgia. For information on these materials and to receive free brochures on related topics, call your local Arthritis Foundation chapter or the national, toll-free line, 800/283-7800. You can also access the Arthritis Foundation Web site at www.arthritis.org.

The Diagnosis Dilemma

Fibromyalgia is a syndrome diagnosed by the identification of symptoms – widespread pain plus tender points – and the exclusion of other conditions. That means undergoing initial laboratory tests to rule out maladies with similar symptoms, such as thyroid conditions.

No evidence of fibromyalgia appears on X-rays or in laboratory test results. There is no diagnostic marker in the blood. People with fibromyalgia often look healthy with no outward signs of pain or fatigue. Diagnosis of children may be especially difficult because they often have trouble describing their symptoms.

For people with fibromyalgia, diagnostic testing can seem endless and exasperating. Despite its prevalence, fibromyalgia remains unfamiliar to many people and even doctors. Medical schools began teaching about the condition only relatively recently. The lack of general knowledge and the scarcity of objective physical evidence for fibromyalgia lead many people on a long and often frustrating quest for answers.

According to Don L. Goldenberg, MD, chief of rheumatology and director of the Arthritis-Fibromyalgia Center at Newton-Wellesley Hospital in Newton, Massachusetts, studies show that most people with fibromyalgia spend an average of five years seeking a diagnosis after they start experiencing symptoms. This pursuit is frustrating at best.

Fortunately, a greater understanding of fibromyalgia now exists within the medical community. Although the underlying cause remains undetermined, new research has uncovered exciting leads and better treatments.

What Causes Fibromyalgia?

Scientists have not determined the cause of fibromyalgia, although a number of theories exist. Some studies show that an injury or trauma, physical or emotional, may affect the central nervous system's response to pain. For example, in 1997, when Israeli researchers compared patients with neck injuries to those with legs injuries, they found that fibromyalgia was 13 times more likely to develop after neck trauma. Other researchers believe hormonal changes or infections, such as a flu virus, may trigger fibromyalgia.

There are some scientists who suspect that lack of exercise and changes in muscle metabolism may play a role in fibromyalgia or that the opposite, muscle overuse, may be the key.

Sleep disturbance, a symptom of fibromyalgia, may also be a cause. Sleep disturbance lowers the production of a growth hormone crucial to the repair of muscles.

An established link exists between fibromyalgia and depression, but no one knows if depression is a cause or effect of the ailment. What does seem to be true is that all of these conditions may contribute to fibromyalgia. Different people appear to get fibromyalgia for different reasons.

For years, a theory held that fibromyalgia may be caused by a defect in how muscles use energy. However, a 1994 study challenged that theory. By measuring muscle energy metabolism, rheumatologist Robert Simms, MD, associate professor of medicine and director of clinical rheumatology at Boston University School of Medicine, and his colleagues were able to show that the muscles of people who have equivalent levels of aerobic fitness use energy in the same way whether they have fibromyalgia or not.

Researchers also are interested in similarities between fibromyalgia and other similar syndromes such as chronic fatigue syndrome, another tenacious condition of unknown origin that also is characterized by muscle pain, poor sleep and persistent fatigue. In the fourth edition of the *Textbook of Rheumatology*, Dr. Bennett devotes a chapter to examining the relation between fibromyalgia, chronic fatigue syndrome and *myofascial pain*, a fibromyalgia-type pain produced by trauma and limited to only one or two parts of the body. Two common forms of myofascial pain include temporomandibular joint disorder, characterized by jaw pain, and *repetitive strain syndrome*, which causes muscle problems associated with repetitive workplace tasks such as typing. Doctors believe the early treatment of these conditions may prevent the onset of full-blown fibromyalgia. Dr. Bennett and others also now believe that fibromyalgia may be at the high end of a spectrum of

chronic pain. This spectrum ranges from short-lived, localized pain at one end to insistent widespread pain and *allodynia,* or pain on light touch, at the other end.

PAIN AND HORMONES

Some researchers theorize that hormones may play a role in fibromyalgia pain. Hormones are substances that are secreted by the body's glands, such as the adrenal glands or the pituitary gland. Hormones have a regulatory effect on different parts of the body.

Neural hormones are one type of hormone, chemical messengers of the central nervous system that affect functions such as sleep, pain sensation, immunity, the constriction and dilation of blood vessels and even emotions.

Think of the central nervous system as a central electrical wiring system for the body. Like wires, neurons carry electrical impulses from the farthest reaches of fingers and toes to the spinal cord, where all the wiring comes together as in your home's circuit-breaker box. Just as the electric company monitors your breaker box through wires, the brain manages the nervous system through spinal cord connections. Within this elaborate system, each hormone has a separate job, but each job influences the others.

Scientists now believe that many people with fibromyalgia may process neural hormones, including serotonin, another hormone called *substance P* and growth hormones differently than other people.

Some researchers purport that the central nervous systems of people with fibromyalgia may process pain differently than the nervous systems of other people. One theory suggests that in fibromyalgia, the nervous system interprets light stimuli, such as the slightest touch or pressure, as painful. This process is called *central sensitization*. What causes this excess sensitivity to ordinary stimuli in people with fibromyalgia? One cause may be the *wind-up phenomena*, a state that occurs when certain nerve fibers, called N-methyl-D-aspartate (NMDA) receptors, are stimulated repeatedly over a long period, increasing the frequency of pain messages to the brain. The brain in turn becomes overactive and perceives light stimuli as painful. It is still unclear whether central sensitization happens as a result of the chronic pain in fibromyalgia, or if central sensitization actually causes fibromyalgia pain. Researchers do not yet know the answer to this question. One possible clue is that some tests have shown that in people with fibromyalgia, blood flow through several parts of the brain – including the cingulate cortex, which interprets the emotional components of pain, and the thalamus, which regulates pain signals – is different than in the brains of people without the condition.

Following are explanations of the different hormones that may play a role in fibromyalgia pain, and what role each may play.

• **Substance P.** When the body is injured, neurons go on red alert, serving as a hotline and surveillance system. The news of the injury reaches the brain at lightning speed. A neural hormone called *substance P* is released in the neurons and in the spinal cord. Its job is to send a loud pain message back to the brain.

Studies have shown that levels of substance P in the spinal cord are three times higher than normal in people with fibromyalgia. One research study conducted by Jon Russell, MD, of the University of Texas Health Sciences Center in San Antonio indicated that spinal fluid levels of substance P in people with fibromyalgia remain consistently high for weeks to months, suggesting a persistent elevation of the neurochemical in the central nervous systems of people with fibromyalgia.

When Dr. Russell applied pressure to the tender points of people with fibromyalgia for approximately five minutes, it did not cause a measurable increase in the spinal fluid substance P levels. The study participants still felt pain because the pressure causes a normal release of pain messengers in the spinal cord, regardless of the already-elevated levels of substance P. The fact that pressure does not further lift substance P levels in the spinal fluid, however, suggests that constantly elevated levels are not simply the result of minor bumps or bruises, nor an abnormality in the skin, muscle or bone. Rather, the constantly elevated levels of hormone may result from an abnormal process in the brain or spinal cord of people with fibromyalgia. This study may suggest that although exercise may be painful, it does not actually damage or permanently injure the muscles.

• **Serotonin.** When pain occurs, the body has a way of turning down the volume on the message. Serotonin, a neurotransmitter that regulates the brain's ability to control pain and mood, is one substance released in the brain and spinal cord to do the job.

Some researchers have found that levels of serotonin may be low or that serotonin may be poorly processed in people with fibromyalgia. Serotonin facilitates deep, restorative sleep. A lack of serotonin may lead to a lack of this deep sleep, and poor sleep is a common symptom in fibromyalgia. Decreases in serotonin may also lead to an alteration in the amount of substance P released with each painful stimulus (thus sending pronounced pain messages to the brain) and lower levels of the stress hormones in the brain that regulate our stress responses.

• **Hypothalamic-pituitary-adrenal (HPA) hormones.** The link between lowered stress hormones, or HPA hormones, and fibromyalgia intrigues researchers because both physical and emotional stress are thought to play a role in the syndrome. A person may feel out of control when confronted with a stressful situation. But the human body has a well-defined set of emergency procedures to deal with stress. The success of these procedures relies on how effectively hormones relay messages to the brain.

One of the most familiar hormones is *adrenaline.* When we are frightened, the body responds with a rush of this hormone. Secreted by the *adrenal glands*, organs located near the kidneys, adrenaline accelerates heart and respiration rates. Adrenaline prepares us to run for our lives or stand and fight the dangerous situation. HPA hormones, secreted by the hypothalamic-pituitary-adrenal axis, are less dramatic but equally essential to survival. HPA hormones

are key stress responders that ensure that the mind can focus and the body can respond properly to stress. People with fibromyalgia may secrete these hormones differently than other people when faced with stress.

When some of her patients associated the onset of their fibromyalgia with intense physical or emotional stress and fluctuations in symptom severity corresponded to levels of daily stress, Leslie Crofford, MD, associate professor of internal medicine at the University of Michigan in Ann Arbor, was intrigued. Dr. Crofford and her research team explored the biological differences between people who can take stress in stride and those people who respond to stress with a painful fibromyalgia flare.

Dr. Crofford's team found that people with fibromyalgia secrete stress hormones differently than others. After their glands are stimulated, people with fibromyalgia secrete more *pituitary hormones*, the hormones that affect energy, and less adrenaline than people without the condition. Dr. Crofford and her colleagues also have found that in people with fibromyalgia, there are differences in the *circadian rhythms* (the internal schedule for the body's biological tasks) that influence hormone secretion.

Normally, hormone secretion is active in the early morning, tapers off during the day, is quiet in the evening. It is activated also as an emergency response to stress. In people with fibromyalgia, however, secretion of pituitary hormones occurs later in the morning than normal, leading to elevated secretions of adrenaline, or stress-related, hormones throughout the day. People with fibromyalgia may have unpleasant mornings due to this delayed secretion of pituitary (or energy-affecting) hormones and elevation of adrenaline throughout the rest of their day.

Our bodies' stress systems are part of what link mind and body responses. Many of the symptoms of fibromyalgia – sleep disturbance, fatigue, difficulty concentrating – are tied to the brain and could influence or be influenced by stress hormones. In addition, our stress responses influence how our brain perceives pain signals. Dr. Crofford also notes that stress can alter blood flow and muscle metabolism, which may point to further connections between an abnormal release of stress hormones and the many symptoms of fibromyalgia.

• **Growth hormones.** Lowered serotonin may not only affect levels of stress hormones. It also may lower the secretion of growth hormones in the body. A decreased level of growth hormones may be connected to the lack of deep, restorative sleep in many people with fibromyalgia.

In 1992, Dr. Bennett and his colleagues at Oregon Health Sciences University linked fibromyalgia to disturbed sleep. Parts of the body, including the liver and probably the kidney, secrete a growth hormone called *somatomedin C.* Essential to the body's task of rebuilding itself, somatomedin C is secreted primarily in the fourth stage of sleep, delta sleep, the deepest and most restorative level of daily sleeping.

Dr. Bennett found that people with fibromyalgia have significantly lower levels of somatomedin C in their blood than those without the condition. Another researcher

with a special interest in this field is Harvey Moldofsky, MD, of the Center for Sleep and Chronobiology at Western Division Toronto Hospital. Dr. Moldofsky and his co-workers, pioneers in the science of *chronobiology*, or the timing of biologic events, demonstrated that when the same sleep abnormality that occurs in deep sleep was induced in people without fibromyalgia, they also developed symptoms of the condition.

Lowered levels of yet another growth hormone, IGF-1, also appear in about one third of people with fibromyalgia. In a 1998 study, Dr. Bennett and his colleagues gave people with fibromyalgia daily injections of growth hormone, and after nine months the group's symptoms and number of tender points diminished.

It is not yet clear how these findings on the connections between hormone and neurochemical disturbances and fibromyalgia will impact the average person living with the syndrome. All of these research trails – Dr. Crofford's work with stress hormones, Dr. Russell's research on serotonin and substance P, and Dr. Bennett's work on growth hormones – may eventually cross on the way to finding a cause or causes of fibromyalgia.

THE MIND-BODY CONNECTION

When emotions and stress are expressed through physical symptoms, the condition is called *somatic* from the Greek word *soma*, meaning body. Fibromyalgia is such a condition. It joins other similar syndromes called *functional somatic syndromes* such as irritable bowel syndrome, chronic fatigue syndrome and Gulf War syndrome (a mysterious illness striking many veterans of the early 1990s conflict). All of these syndromes are characterized by symptoms such as headaches, painful muscles, fatigue and insomnia and a higher rate of psychiatric symptoms. In fact, it's not unusual for people with one syndrome to have one or more of the others.

Some doctors speculate that these syndromes all involve some kind of flaw in the body's nervous system and its response to stress. Although doctors aren't certain why the flaw occurs, they do recognize that emotions influence our bodies. Stress, as we have seen in the preceding section, affects our hormones, which in turn affect our bodies and the way they function.

Although everyone's body is affected by emotion, some people have a stronger reaction than others. Some people may have family and friends who reinforce their idea of themselves as sick. Or they may be experiencing other life traumas, such as divorce or the loss of a loved one, which may disturb sleep or lead to depression. Divorce and disturbed sleep may then reinforce the symptoms of the illness. Because emotions and stressful situations may influence hormone secretion and other bodily functions, they can be especially difficult for someone with fibromyalgia.

THE GENETIC CONNECTION

Fibromyalgia may occur in several members of the same family, but many doctors believe common environmental factors could be the cause rather than genetic factors. In 1998, however, Dr. Yunus and his colleagues at the University of Illinois College of Medicine found a possible link between certain human leukocyte antigens (HLAs) and fibromyalgia. They also found a link between HLAs and depression, commonly associated with fibromyalgia. Although researchers are cautious about interpreting the findings, they are the strongest suggestion to date of a genetic basis for fibromyalgia.

FIBROMYALGIA AND THE GULF WAR SYNDROME

War-related syndromes date back to the Civil War and perhaps earlier. Following the 1991 Persian Gulf War, 3,000 soldiers reported persistent symptoms such as fatigue and joint pain two to three months after the war. According to at least one study of Gulf War veterans, 17 percent of its subjects had fibromyalgia. Less than two percent of the total U.S. population has fibromyalgia, so this incidence of the syndrome is high. Although doctors aren't certain of the connection, they do believe this syndrome may be more evidence that stress and trauma trigger fibromyalgia.

FIBROMYALGIA AND SEXUAL ABUSE

Researchers also have explored a possible link between physical and emotional trauma, such as sexual abuse, and fibromyalgia. In 1995, two studies were published in *Arthritis & Rheumatism,* a scholarly journal published by the American College of Rheumatology, on the prevalence of sexual and physical abuse in women with fibromyalgia syndrome. In that same journal, James I. Hudson, MD, and Harrison G. Pope Jr., MD, published an editorial exploring whether or not childhood sexual abuse was a possible cause of fibromyalgia. Although there may be an association between sexual abuse and the number and severity of symptoms related to fibromyalgia, neither study concluded that sexual abuse is a cause.

Researchers do seem to agree that physical and sexual abuse seem to be associated with a range of chronic pain syndromes, including fibromyalgia. However, the number of fibromyalgia patients with a history of either type of abuse is relatively small.

Chapter 2

Relieving Symptoms:

Treatments for Fibromyalgia

Although fibromyalgia has no known cure, its symptoms can be treated through a variety of approaches, from drugs to relaxation techniques to simply avoiding activities that may worsen symptoms. In the following two chapters, we will discuss the most common treatments for the many, varied symptoms of fibromyalgia.

Treatment: Multiple Options

People with fibromyalgia may find benefit from a care program that includes some or all of the following suggestions:

• moderate exercise, to stretch muscles and improve cardiovascular fitness
• relaxation techniques, to reduce stress
• education, to help people understand and cope with the condition
• healthy habits, such as eating well and not smoking
• medications to diminish pain and improve sleep
• alternative therapies such as acupuncture, massage, or herbs and supplements

Each of these techniques will be discussed in depth in individual chapters, but the following overview introduces them, allowing you to decide which treatments you'd like to learn more about and to compare these to your own regimen.

Many people with fibromyalgia are able to manage their symptoms with some lifestyle changes, such as adjustments in daily goals, diet, exercise and over-the-counter nonsteroidal anti-inflammatory drugs (NSAIDs), such as aspirin, ibuprofen (*Advil*) or naproxen sodium (*Aleve*), and analgesics, such as acetaminophen (*Tylenol*). Many others, however, take prescription medications, including antidepressants such as tricyclics and specific serotonin reuptake inhibitors (SSRIs) like fluoxetine (*Prozac*) and sertraline (*Zoloft*). However, studies of SSRIs and fibromyalgia have shown mixed results. Although they may help some people, SSRIs also may interrupt sleep, an obviously unhelpful side effect. No drug specifically has been approved by the Food and Drug Administration for treating fibromyalgia, but there are many drugs that doctors can prescribe for people with the condition.

Children with fibromyalgia, however, often are treated with exercise therapy, which is frequently paired with psychological treatment. Over-the-counter medications or prescription medications such as antidepressants may be prescribed by a doctor for children with fibromyalgia. The Arthritis Foundation is funding research to determine which treatments are appropriate for children or adolescents.

EXERCISE AND PHYSICAL THERAPY

Regular exercise can help anyone feel better, but people with fibromyalgia can especially reap enormous benefits. Toned, well-conditioned muscles can diminish the pain of fibromyalgia, and aerobic fitness can improve sleep. Exercise also raises levels of serotonin and endorphins (see Chapter 1), both of which boost moods and lessen pain.

People with fibromyalgia may be reluctant to exercise if they are tired and in pain. Low- or non-impact aerobic exercises such as walking, biking, swimming or water aerobics are a few types of exercise that may not overtax painful muscles. Regular workouts of gradually increased frequency and duration will improve fitness. Gently stretching muscles before and after your workout will increase exercise endurance. Chapter 6 presents a more in-depth look at exercise and its benefits for people with fibromyalgia.

Doctors also may prescribe physical therapy, which can include a specific exercise program, and such pain-management treatments such as heat, ice, massage, whirlpool, ultrasound, electrical nerve stimulation and biofeedback.

REST AND RELAXATION

In a hectic world, it's often difficult to take time out for rest. But it's important for people with fibromyalgia to do just that. Rest and relaxation (both physical and mental) allow the body time to heal itself, breaking the vicious cycle of pain, stress and depression. Everyone, particularly people with fibromyalgia, needs to balance periods of activity with periods of rest. Chapter 13 presents information about relaxation techniques such as cognitive behavioral therapy, yoga and meditation.

EDUCATION

People with fibromyalgia can be their own best researchers and advocates. By learning about the condition and taking an active role in their care, they can lead healthy lives. Reading this book and any other reliable material about fibromyalgia is a good first step. Ask your doctor questions to help you understand your fibromyalgia and create a dialogue. Seek out support groups and classes to find peers with your condition, or join activity groups such as meditation and yoga classes to boost your knowledge and coping skills. To learn about fibromyalgia support groups or educational programs in your area, contact your local chapter of the Arthritis Foundation by calling 800/283-7800.

Personally Speaking

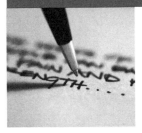

"**M**edicine is a powerful thing. It not only controls how you feel physically but can also control how you think. How do I know this? Because over the past six years, I have dealt with and taken powerful medicine daily.

Making Peace With Medications
Anne DeYoung
Crestwood, Ill

"At 12, I was diagnosed with fibromyalgia and rheumatoid arthritis. At 13, I experienced a flare of both conditions. My doctor put me on high doses of prednisone, a steroid, and I gained a lot of weight. At 13, this is not a good thing. It only took one medicine to depress me so much that I refused to get out of bed. But inactivity caused my flare to become worse, and I needed even higher doses of steroids. I lived in my own vicious circle. And I couldn't stand how I looked. I thought I would never get better.

"My family supported, encouraged and helped me get back on my feet, a process that took about seven months. Finally, I was well enough to get out of bed in the morning or go shopping or get to school. It still amazes me how just one drug could change my outlook on life. I'm still self-conscious about my weight, which I never used to be. Of course, some medicines can make you feel good, too. The muscle relaxants I take after a long, hard day sure make me feel good.

"Staying positive while battling this change in your life can be hard to do, especially if you are feeling alone or scared. I look at pictures of me and my friends or family, call a buddy and talk for hours, take a soothing bath, or just relax in a room with candles and soft music — all simple things you can do without stressing your body.

"I hope my experiences and advice will help at least one person who suffers from fibromyalgia. Attitude and positive thinking are key factors in dealing with life's harsh realities. Try to look forward, never back. You never know what the future may bring."

HEALTHY HABITS

Pain and depression can lead some people with fibromyalgia to eat poorly or seek relief in cigarettes or alcohol, which may worsen symptoms. Giving up unhealthy habits like drinking and smoking allows the body to devote its energy to recovery. Replacing a junky, fast-food diet with a healthy one not only will help someone with fibromyalgia feel better, but it also will ensure that their bodies get the fuel and vitamins they need to battle their condition.

Medications for Fibromyalgia

While self-management techniques such as regular exercise, relaxation and a healthy diet may be the most important methods for tackling fibromyalgia, there are a number of medications available that may offer substantive relief for many of the condition's symptoms.

TRICYCLIC ANTIDEPRESSANTS

Traditionally used for treating depression, tricyclic antidepressants in small dosages can also be effective in treating fibromyalgia. Although most often used for treating depression, tricyclics also relax muscles and increase restorative delta-wave sleep that is often disturbed in people with fibromyalgia.

Restored sleep means greater production of the growth hormones essential to muscle repair, hormones produced only during delta sleep. Tricyclics also increase the amount of serotonin, the hormone important for regulating pain and deep sleep discussed in Chapter 1, available to the nerve cells, and raise the efficiency of *endorphins* (a chemical released by the body when we exercise or laugh). Both serotonin and endorphins are natural painkillers. Serotonin, often found in lower-than-normal levels in people with fibromyalgia, affects sleep and mood.

By promoting sleep, easing pain and relaxing muscles, tricyclics can help some people with fibromyalgia break out of the chronic pain/fatigue symptom cycle. However, studies in which tricyclics were used to treat fibromyalgia have had mixed results. Some show no effect; some show improved sleep and less pain, and some show improvement over the short term. No drug has the same level of effectiveness for every person, but if a person suffers from chronic pain and other symptoms of fibromyalgia, trying a drug that has seen mixed results in studies may be worthwhile.

Examples of tricyclic antidepressants include amitriptyline (*Elavil*), doxepin (*Sinequan*) and nortriptyline (*Pamelor*). Results vary from person to person. Possible side effects include daytime drowsiness, constipation, dry mouth, increased appetite and weight gain.

SSRIS (SELECTIVE SEROTONIN RE-UPTAKE INHIBITORS)

Researchers believe that people with fibromyalgia either have low levels of serotonin or are unable to process it properly. In the mid-1980s, antidepressants called selective serotonin re-uptake inhibitors, or SSRIs, were developed. These drugs aid the release of serotonin, reducing fatigue, mental confusion, depression and pain. Examples of SSRIs include fluoxetine (*Prozac*), sertraline (*Zoloft*) and paroxetine (*Paxil*). As with tricyclics, when SSRIs are used for fibromyalgia, lower dosages can be used than when treating depression.

However, the results of studies on SSRIs' effectiveness have been mixed. In some patients felt less pain. But in others SSRIs showed no more effect than a placebo, or inactive substitute. SSRIs also can have side effects, including insomnia, an effect that may worsen fibromyalgia symptoms.

COMBINATION TREATMENT

In many people with chronic illnesses, a combination of drugs can be more effective than a single drug for treating symptoms, Possibly due to the fact that many chronic illnesses have several, varied symptoms and an unclear cause. A combination of drugs attacks these varied symptoms and helps to improve well-being. Combination treatment also may be effective for fibromyalgia.

In a 1996 study of 19 people with fibromyalgia, researchers at the Newton-Wellesley Hospital in Newton, Massachusetts found that SSRIs used in combination with tricyclics yielded better results than either medication taken alone. Lead researcher Don Goldenberg, MD, reported that although patients improved on either drug, they experienced a 25 percent improvement in pain, fatigue and sleep after six weeks of a combined dose.

NONSTEROIDAL ANTI-INFLAMMATORY DRUGS (NSAIDS)

Nonsteroidal anti-inflammatory drugs, known as NSAIDs, include common drugs such as aspirin, ibuprofen and naproxen. These drugs are available over the counter and in higher dosages by prescription. This group of drugs relieves pain by inhibiting *prostaglandins*, hormone-like acids that control certain body functions, including pain from inflammation.

Inflammation is not a symptom of fibromyalgia, however, so these medications don't have a major effect on the condition. Yet moderate doses may help relieve pain and stiffness. They also may have side effects, including stomach upset and peptic ulcers. NSAIDs have no effect on muscle spasms and cramping other than minor pain relief.

A new class of NSAIDs, called COX-2 specific inhibitors, may be more promising than traditional NSAIDs, in part, because they appear to be easier on the stomach. These drugs include celecoxib (*Celebrex*) and rofecoxib (*Vioxx*). Unlike traditional NSAIDs, these drugs inhibit only COX-2 prostaglandins, which help cause inflammation. Traditional NSAIDs block both COX-1 and COX-2 prostaglandins. COX-1 is a prostaglandin that protects the digestive system from its own acids. When COX-1 prostaglandins are inhibited by drugs, that protection is removed, and the result is often stomach upset.

Because, like their cousins, COX-2 drugs primarily fight inflammation, it's not yet clear how effective they will be for pain in fibromyalgia, which is not caused by inflammation.

ANALGESICS

Analgesics are a group of drugs that relieve pain. Analgesics include over-the-counter varieties and stronger, prescription drugs, such as narcotics. Following are some of the common analgesics used to fight fibromyalgia pain.

• **Acetaminophen.** Acetaminophen is a common, over-the-counter analgesic (the best-known brand is *Tylenol*) that is useful for

The Narcotics Debate

Some doctors would never prescribe narcotics for fibromyalgia. Others argue that they can be an appropriate drug for pain relief and promoting sleep. Even doctors who support their use agree that narcotics are necessary only for a small number of people with fibromyalgia and then only in tandem with a treatment program that includes exercise, education, medications for helping sleep and depression and counseling on lifestyle changes.

If pain relief is not achieved with NSAIDs, tricyclics, acetaminophen or tramadol, then narcotics such as codeine, hydrocodone, oxycodone or methadone may be considered for some people. The decision to go this route requires patient counseling on dependency and expected side effects. Most physicians will require their patients to sign a contract that outlines appropriate use of the drugs and the physician's expectations regarding ongoing use. Below are what many doctors view as central issues in the debate:

Advantages:
• Narcotics are the most effective available medications for managing chronic pain.
• The majority of fibromyalgia patients don't need narcotics. But those who do should have the option for a trial period.
• The addiction rate from narcotics is one percent. Addiction (compulsive, self-destructive use) is not the same as dependence (withdrawal symptoms if the drug is stopped abruptly).
• Less pain results in better functioning.

Disadvantages:
• When you use narcotics, you are treating pain solely as a symptom without necessarily eliminating the factors that cause it. Therefore, narcotics should be used only in the context of a thorough medical management program.
• Dependence is an expected result of treatment.
• Narcotics will dull pain but not eliminate it. In other words, they are not a cure for fibromyalgia.
• Tolerance to narcotics occurs after a time – from months to years – so that increasing the dosage is necessary to maintain the same level of response.
• Narcotics have side effects such as mental fuzziness, constipation, nausea, drowsiness and itching, all of which may be amplified in people with fibromyalgia.

those who wish to avoid aspirin and other NSAIDs. As with NSAIDs, acetaminophen only provides minor relief from fibromyalgia pain and stiffness. Acetaminophen also can damage the liver when taken over a long period with other substances potentially harmful to the liver, such as alcohol.

• **Tramadol hydrochloride.** Tramadol hydrochloride (*Ultram*) is a prescription pain reliever. Tramadol has a slight potential for dependence. It acts by raising serotonin and noradrenaline levels and by blocking several pain pathways, including the NMDA receptor, which as noted earlier may play a part in fibromyalgia pain. Tramadol's possible side effects include nervousness, anxiety and sleep disorder, all of which could worsen fibromyalgia symptoms.

• **Narcotics.** Narcotics are potent drugs that interrupt pain signals traveling to the brain by imitating the body's own endorphins, which block pain signals naturally. Examples of narcotics include propoxyphene hydrochloride (*Darvon*), codeine (often mixed with acetaminophen), hydrocodone (*Vicodin*), demerol and morphine. Narcotics are appropriate only for a small percentage of people with fibromyalgia. Some doctors do not think people with fibromyalgia should use narcotics for pain relief at all due to the risk of dependence on the drugs (see the sidebar).

GLUCOCORTICOIDS

Used to treat some inflammatory forms of arthritis such as rheumatoid arthritis and lupus, glucocorticoids (examples are cortisone and prednisone) are powerful anti-inflammatory agents. These drugs are steroids but not the anabolic steroids used by athletes to bulk up muscles. Glucocorticoid drugs fight inflammation and can have dramatic results.

As inflammation is not a problem in fibromyalgia, glucocorticoids offer little relief for fibromyalgia symptoms, such as pain. According to a 1998 study at the National Institutes of Health, the benefit of pain relief offered by a glucocorticoid called hydrocortisone was offset by a dangerous suppression of the adrenal glands, the glands near the kidneys that secrete a variety of hormones (including adrenaline – see Chapter 1).

Glucocorticoids, sometimes called corticosteroids, also carry a risk of side effects such as weight gain and mood swings. These side effects can be minimized when the drugs are taken in very small dosages.

BENZODIAZEPINES

Benzodiazepines are tranquilizers that can help reduce painful muscle tension and improve sleep. However, they can be addictive if used for long periods. Your physician should monitor your use of tranquilizers, which include drugs such as clonazepam (*Klonopin*), diazepam (*Valium*), diazepoxide (*Librium*) and alprazolam (*Xanax*). These drugs exert a calming effect. Generally, however, tranquilizers are not used for fibromyalgia. Doctors may prescribe a sedative like zolpidem tartrate (*Ambien*) when sleep is a major problem and other approaches to improving sleep have not helped.

TENDER-POINT INJECTIONS

A local anesthetic directly injected into a patient's tender points can provide relief that lasts from hours to several months. These injections are initially painful and generally used only in cases of severe or persistent tender-point pain.

TOPICAL OINTMENTS

Topical ointments are applied directly to the skin on the areas where pain occurs. A variety of brands of topical ointments are available over the counter. Some ointments contain a deep-heating ingredient called *methyl salicylate* that may increase blood flow to the skin, soothing painful muscles. Other creams containing *capsaicin,* the fiery oil in chili peppers, may be used to modify joint pain or nerve pain temporarily. Capsaicin works by decreasing the ability of nerve endings in the skin to sense pain. However, capsaicin products may not be practical management tools for fibromyalgia pain, because the ointments must be applied two or three times a day, and because the areas affected by fibromyalgia are so extensive.

For more comprehensive information about drugs for treating the symptoms of fibromyalgia, contact the Arthritis Foundation at 800/283-7800 and request a free copy of the 2001 Drug Guide. Or, visit www.arthritis.org and view the Drug Guide online.

Drugs Used in Treating Fibromyalgia

At this time, there are no drugs specifically approved by the Food and Drug Administration for treating fibromyalgia. Here are some drugs that may alleviate certain symptoms associated with fibromyalgia, including pain, sleep problems and muscle aches.

ANALGESICS

These are drugs used for pain relief. Other than acetaminophen, these have the potential for dependence if used for long periods of time.

Acetaminophen
Brand names: *Anacin (aspirin-free), Excedrin caplets, Panadol, Tylenol*
Dosage: 325 to 1,000 mg every 4 to 6 hours as needed, no more than 3,000 mg per day
Possible side effects: When taken as prescribed, acetaminophen is usually not associated with side effects.

Acetaminophen with codeine
Brand names: *Fioricet, Phenaphen with codeine, Tylenol with codeine*
Dosage: 15 to 60 mg codeine every 4 hours as needed
Possible side effects: Constipation, dizziness or lightheadedness, drowsiness, nausea, unusual tiredness or weakness, vomiting

Hydrocodone with acetaminophen
Brand names: *Dolacet, Hydrocet, Lorcet, Lortab, Vicodin*
Dosage: 2.5 to 10 mg hydrocodone every 4 to 6 hours as needed
Possible side effects: Dizziness, drowsiness, lightheadedness or feeling faint, nausea or vomiting, unusual tiredness or weakness

Oxycodone
Brand names: *OxyContin, Roxicodone*
Dosage: For OxyContin, 10 mg every 12 hours as needed; for Roxicodone, 5 mg every 3 to 6 hours or 10 mg 3 or 4 times a day as needed
Possible side effects: Dizziness, drowsiness, lightheadedness or feeling faint, nausea or vomiting, unusual tiredness or weakness

Propoxyphene hydrochloride
Brand names: *Darvon, PC-Cap, Wygesic*
Dosage: 65 mg every 4 hours as needed, no more than 390 mg per day
Possible side effects: Dizziness or lightheadedness, drowsiness, nausea and vomiting

Tramadol
Brand name: *Ultram*
Dosage: 50 to 100 mg every 6 hours as needed
Possible side effects: Dizziness, nausea, constipation, headache, sleepiness

Drugs Used in Treating Fibromyalgia (cont.)

ANTIDEPRESSANTS

Antidepressants, including tricyclics and selective serotonin reuptake inhibitors (SSRIs), help people with fibromyalgia get the deep, restorative sleep they often lack. These drugs are taken in smaller doses than they are when used to treat depression.

Tricyclics:
Amitriptyline hydrochloride
Brand name: *Elavil, Endep*
Dosage: 10 to 80 mg per day in a single dose
Possible side effects: Difficulty concentrating, dizziness, drowsiness, dry mouth, headache, increased appetite (including craving for sweets), nausea, sleep disturbances, unpleasant taste, urinary retention, weakness or tiredness, weight gain

Doxepin
Brand name: *Adapin, Sinequan*
Dosage: 10 to 100 mg per day a few hours before bedtime in a single dose
Possible side effects: Difficulty concentrating, dizziness, drowsiness, dry mouth, headache, increased appetite (including craving for sweets), nausea, sleep disturbances, unpleasant taste, urinary retention, weakness or tiredness, weight gain

Nortriptyline
Brand name: *Aventyl, Pamelor*
Dosage: 10 to 100 mg per day a few hours before bedtime in a single dose
Possible side effects: Difficulty concentrating, dizziness, drowsiness, dry mouth, headache, increased appetite (including craving for sweets), nausea, sleep disturbances, unpleasant taste, urinary retention, weakness or tiredness, weight gain

Selective Serotonin Reuptake Inhibitors (SSRIs)
Fluoxetine
Brand name: *Prozac*
Dosage: 20 to 80 mg per day in a single dose
Possible side effects: Anxiety and nervousness, diarrhea, dry mouth, headache, increased sweating, nausea, trouble sleeping

Paroxetine
Brand name: *Paxil*
Dosage: 10 to 60 mg per day in a single dose
Possible side effects: Constipation, decreased sexual ability, dizziness, dry mouth, headache, nausea, difficulty urinating, tremors, trouble sleeping, unusual tiredness or weakness, vomiting

Sertraline
Brand name: *Zoloft*
Dosage: 25 to 200 mg per day in a single dose
Possible side effects: Decreased appetite or weight loss; decreased sexual drive or ability; diarrhea; drowsiness; dryness of the mouth; headache, stomach or abdominal cramps, gas or pain; tremors; trouble sleeping; clumsiness or unsteadiness; dizziness or lightheadedness; drowsiness; slurred speech

BENZODIAZEPINES - SLEEP MEDICATION

Temazepam
Brand name: *Restoril*
Dosage: 15 mg per day in a single dose
Possible side effects: When taken as prescribed, temazepam is not usually associated with side effects.

MUSCLE RELAXANTS

Cyclobenzaprine
Brand names: *Cycloflex, Flexeril*
Dosage: 10 to 40 mg per day best tolerated as a single dose several hours before bedtime
Possible side effects: Dizziness or lightheadedness, drowsiness, dry mouth, confusion

OTHER DRUGS USED FOR FIBROMYALGIA

Maprotiline
Brand names: *Ludiomil*
Dosage: 25 to 150 mg per day in 1 to 3 doses
Possible side effects: Blurred vision, decreased sexual ability, dizziness or lightheadedness, drowsiness, dry mouth, headaches, increased or decreased sexual drive, tiredness or weakness

Trazodone
Brand names: *Desyrel, Trazon, Trialodine*
Dosage: 50 to 150 mg per day in 2 or 3 doses
Possible side effects: Dizziness or lightheadedness, drowsiness, dry mouth, headache, nausea and vomiting, unpleasant taste in mouth

Zolpidem
Brand names: *Ambien*
Dosage: 10 mg per day in a single dose
Possible side effects: Side effects are uncommon at prescribed dosage.

Drugs Used in Treating Fibromyalgia (cont.)

NSAIDS: NONSTEROIDAL ANTI-INFLAMMATORY DRUGS

NSAIDs reduce inflammation, which is not a feature of fibromyalgia, but some people with fibromyalgia may take over-the-counter NSAIDs for mild pain relief.

Note: Possible side effects for all NSAIDs, except where noted, include abdominal pain, fluid retention, gastric ulcers and bleeding, greater susceptibility to bruising or bleeding from cuts, heartburn, indigestion, lightheadedness, nausea, reduction in kidney function, increase in liver enzymes. COX-2 inhibitors, a new class of NSAID, are less likely to cause gastrointestinal distress or stomach ulcers. If you consume more than three alcoholic drinks per day, check with your doctor before using these products.

Aspirin
Brand names: *Anacin, Ascriptin, Bayer, Bufferin, Ecotrin, Excedrin Tablets, ZORprin, others*
Dosage: 3,600 to 5,400 mg per day in several doses

Ibuprofen
Brand names: *Advil, Motrin, Motrin IB, Mediprin, Nuprin*
Dosage: 200 to 400 mg every 4 to 6 hours as needed, not exceeding 1,200 mg per day

Ketoprofen
Brand names: *Actron, Orudis KT*
Dosage: 12.5 mg every 4 to 6 hours as needed

Naproxen sodium
Brand names: *Aleve*
Dosage: 220 mg every 8 to 12 hours as needed

COX-2 INHIBITORS – PRESCRIPTION ONLY

Celecoxib
Brand names: *Celebrex*
Dosage: 200 mg per day in 1 or 2 doses

Rofecoxib
Brand names: *Vioxx*
Dosage: 12.5 mg or 25 mg per day in a single dose

Chapter 3

Alternative Therapies:

Treatment's Old and New Frontier

By working with your doctor, you will determine an overall treatment plan for fibromyalgia that meets your specific needs. Your doctor may prescribe any of the drugs discussed in Chapter 2, but there are many nondrug treatments and alternative therapies that may help control your symptoms as well. Some components of your fibromyalgia treatment — such as exercise, which we'll discuss fully in Chapter 6 — have been proven to be effective at helping reduce pain and fatigue. Others, such as acupuncture, herbal dietary supplements and yoga, may offer pain relief, but it is difficult to determine their true effectiveness for fibromyalgia.

In this chapter, we will explain what *alternative and complementary therapies* are, how they may affect the symptoms of your fibromyalgia, and how you can be a proactive, cautious consumer of these therapies.

Alternative and Complementary Therapies

Over the past several years, many people have become interested in alternative and complementary therapies. The reasons for this interest range from inadequate relief obtained from traditional therapies to the appeal of treatments made of natural ingredients.

Until recently, the term *alternative medicine* was used to describe all therapies outside of mainstream Western medicine used to treat various ailments. Now the more common term is *complementary therapies*, which refers to unconventional treatments used in conjunction with a traditional treatment plan.

Ironically, many of the alternative therapies predate the so-called traditional treatments by centuries. But their acceptance by mainstream medicine is relatively recent.

Complementary therapies may:
• ease some symptoms, such as pain, fatigue, stress and depression
• improve your outlook and attitude

- work in tandem with your conventional therapies to enhance the effects of both.

You should not expect complementary therapies to replace completely the rest of your treatment plan or cure your fibromyalgia. Instead consider these therapies to be something additional you may choose to do for yourself to take control of your condition.

Approach alternative therapies with caution and only with the approval of your doctor. Although many of these therapies are promising, a large number have not been scientifically tested for safety or effectiveness. Some alternative remedies are even fraudulent and have no scientific basis. Others are new treatments that are still under study.

Alternative remedies are considered unproven or experimental until repeated, controlled, scientific studies show they work and won't cause dangerous side effects. Examples of unproven remedies often used for treating fibromyalgia include *St. John's wort,* an herbal supplement, and *acupuncture,* an ancient Chinese medical practice explained later in this chapter.

Some unproven remedies are harmless, but some are not. Even a harmless therapy can hurt you if it causes you to stop or slow down other helpful treatments prescribed by your doctor. Don't take a supplement that does the same thing as a prescribed drug you are taking. In other words, do not take St. John's wort for your depression if you're also taking *Prozac,* because both substances can raise serotonin levels. Raising serotonin levels too high or too rapidly can have harmful side

effects such as tremors, anxiety and even prostration (utter physical or mental exhaustion).

Always be sure to discuss whatever complementary therapies you're trying with your doctor. Discussing these therapies gives your doctor the opportunity to keep an eye out for any dangers or side effects you may experience. For in-depth information on more than 90 alternative and complementary therapies for all types of arthritis, consult *The Arthritis*

Learn More About Alternative Therapies

The Arthritis Foundation's Guide to Alternative Therapies ($24.95) offers reliable answers to your questions about nearly 90 different forms of alternative treatments for arthritis, including supplements, acupuncture, tai chi, yoga, chiropractic, meditation, magnet therapy and more. To order the book, call 800/207-8633 or visit the Arthritis Foundation's online arthritis store at www.arthritis.org.

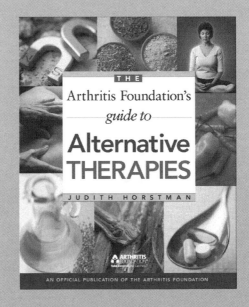

THE

Arthritis Foundation's
guide to

Alternative
THERAPIES

JUDITH HORSTMAN

AN OFFICIAL PUBLICATION OF THE ARTHRITIS FOUNDATION

Foundation's Guide to Alternative Therapies (see box on previous page).

ACUPUNCTURE AND ACUPRESSURE

Many fibromyalgia patients try acupuncture, a Chinese practice of puncturing the body with needles at specific points to relieve pain. The practice is based on the Chinese theory of *qi*, which holds that energy flows throughout the body along 14 invisible pathways called *meridians*. The places where these pathways surface on the skin are called *acupuncture points*.

Acupuncture sessions normally last 30 minutes to an hour, but at the first session the practitioner may spend a little longer with you to ask questions about your overall health, diet, sleep and other habits. Your treatment also may include suggestions about lifestyle and diet.

For the actual acupuncture treatment, the practitioner will insert up to 15 thin needles (they should be sterile and disposable) at specific points of the body that relate to the source of your pain. According to the philosophy of Chinese medicine, these acupuncture points may not be where you feel the pain. For example, the practitioner may treat back pain by pricking points in the feet. Both the place where you feel pain and the place where the acupuncturist pricks may be at different points of the same meridian. Sometimes an acupuncturist combines the needle treatments with heat or gentle electric stimulation.

Acupuncture is a source of skepticism for many Western physicians because the concepts of qi and meridians do not correspond to their understanding of the human anatomy. Therefore, they have no explanation for why acupuncture does, in fact, provide relief to some people. One theory, however, is that when trigger points are stimulated by acupuncture, the body's pain-killing chemicals, such as endorphins or serotonin, are released.

Many doctors think that acupuncture, if done by an experienced practitioner, is safe and possibly effective. A review of seven studies done on acupuncture and fibromyalgia indicates that acupuncture helps relieve pain and stiffness and improves sleep. However, only one of the studies was a high-quality study, so more are needed to confirm its effectiveness. Many doctors believe that acupuncture works best in partnership with other treatments, such as drug therapy.

Acupressure is similar to acupuncture, except practitioners apply pressure on specific points with their fingers or with tools instead of with needles. As with acupuncture, acupressure may not work, and even less is known about its effectiveness than about acupuncture.

Both acupuncture and acupressure practitioners are certified in many states and by several national organizations. To find an acupuncture or acupressure professional, ask your doctor for a recommendation, or contact the National Certification Commission for Acupuncture and Oriental Medicine at 703/548-9004 or www.nccaom.org.

MASSAGE

Massage is a way of handling the body's soft tissues using pressure and stroking. There are many kinds of massage, but the most common is Swedish or European massage, which involves hand-kneading the top layers of muscles, often using oils or lotions. Other types include deep tissue massage (pressure on muscle layers to relieve tension), trigger-point massage (pressure on specific knots of tension), and acupressure massage (as described in the preceding section). Studies show that massage can decrease stress hormones, depression and muscle pain, increase endorphin levels, and improve sleep and immune function.

Massage may offer only temporary pain relief, and you may have to have several therapy sessions before you have noticeable results.

Massage involves pressure, but it should not cause pain. Speak to your massage therapist if you feel pain. People with fibromyalgia may wish to avoid vigorous or deep-tissue massage, which could be painful for them, and opt for Swedish or trigger-point massage instead.

Your doctor can recommend qualified massage therapists in your area, and there are often local organizations that list reputable professionals. Ask a massage therapist these questions before you choose to schedule your treatment:

• Is the therapist certified or licensed by a state board or accreditation agency? If not, look for one who is licensed.

• Does the therapist have any experience with fibromyalgia and your special physical needs? If not, find a therapist who is familiar with your condition.

• Does the therapist claim that massage therapy can cure your fibromyalgia? If so, look for another therapist – this is a false claim.

• Can the therapy be performed in your home? Many massage therapists do offer this service, and it may be more convenient and comfortable for you.

• Does the therapist listen to your concerns? If there is no open dialogue between you, find another therapist.

BIOFEEDBACK

Biofeedback is a therapy that helps you learn to relax muscle tension. This method has the best results when combined with relaxation and other mind-body techniques. In fibromyalgia, muscles often are tense due to pain, so they may contract or tighten after activity instead of relaxing like muscles normally do. Biofeedback helps teach people with fibromyalgia to control their muscles and make them relax, relieving fatigue and pain.

In biofeedback, electronic instruments are attached to the body to measure various physical functions such as pulse and blood pressure. By practicing relaxation techniques and watching how the body reacts via the electronic monitor, people can learn to control body responses to relieve conditions such as chronic pain, muscle tension and stress. Biofeedback may help them develop a better awareness of how to use and control their muscles.

Although in the past doctors were skeptical about biofeedback, many studies since have shown it to be a safe and effective treatment. The timing of results varies from individual to individual, but in most cases, six to 10 biofeedback sessions allow you to learn the necessary muscle-control techniques. As with any therapy, speak to your doctor before you engage in biofeedback to see if it's right for you. With a physician referral, your insurance may cover the therapy. Chapter 13 has more information on biofeedback.

YOGA

Yoga is an ancient Indian practice involving specific exercises, meditation and breathing techniques – a true mind/body activity. When combined with relaxation techniques, yoga may promote flexibility and pain relief, alleviate depression, increase alertness and improve sleep. It's easy to recognize that yoga's potential health benefits would complement fibromyalgia treatments. Yoga is a gentle exercise method that's not too extreme for people with fibromyalgia. (Exercise is discussed more fully in Chapter 6. There is more information on yoga's specific benefits for stress relief in Chapter 13.)

Yoga involves gentle muscle stretching and repetitive, flowing motions that aid flexibility and strength. Breathing and meditation (explained later in this chapter) allow the body and mind to relax, easing tension.

There are different types of yoga, but most Americans practice *Hatha* yoga, which emphasizes body control. More strenuous types of yoga that involve rigorous aerobic activity or extreme contortion should be avoided by people with fibromyalgia.

Stick to gentle movements and relaxation techniques. Hatha yoga is taught by qualified instructors at many health clubs and community centers, so ask your doctor to recommend a course or instructor. You can also contact the American Yoga Association at 941/927-4977 for more information.

Other Techniques for Reducing Pain and Stress

There are many techniques that people with fibromyalgia may explore in order to reduce their pain and stress. Among these methods are meditation, including Transcendental Meditation (TM), hypnosis, and guided imagery or visualization. Reputable studies show that these techniques, particularly in conjunction with traditional treatments, can have a beneficial effect on symptoms such as stress, depression and pain. At the very least, these methods have virtually no side effects, and they can aid relaxation and enhance physical and psychological well-being. There is more information on the benefits of each of these techniques, plus guided imagery exercises you can try, in Chapter 13.

MEDITATION

Meditation is a practice of focused concentration and relaxation. Meditation may take the form of prayer, or it may mean controlled breathing and deep concentration practiced in Eastern meditation. One of the best-known of these forms of meditation is Transcendental Meditation, popularized by the Beatles, Mia Farrow and other celebrities in the 1960s. Meditation can be done with the help of an instructor, or you can create your own method.

Meditation can be as simple as sitting in a quiet place and concentrating on a word, phrase (known as a *mantra*), thought or object. The meditator may modulate her breathing in order to promote a relaxed state. Practice makes perfect in meditation. Mastering the ability to stay still and concentrate may take a while.

A number of uncontrolled studies have suggested that frequent, consistent meditation by fibromyalgia patients alleviates some pain and stress. But more controlled, scientific studies are needed to ascertain meditation's true medical benefits. Regardless, meditation can be a relaxing experience, and a much-needed quiet period for people with fibromyalgia.

HYPNOSIS

Hypnosis is an ancient practice that first attracted notice for its healing potential in the late 18th century when Austrian physician Franz Anton Mesmer used the technique on his patients. The term *mesmerism,* derived from his name, is another term for hypnosis. Despite its prevalence in magic shows, hypnosis is often a useful element in psychotherapy and as a way to promote relaxation and stop unhealthy behaviors, such as smoking.

In hypnotism, a practitioner helps the patient enter a deeply relaxed state. Then, he or she offers suggestions such as that the person's pain or anxiety is subsiding. It's believed that in a hypnotic state, a person is aware of what is going on but is relaxed enough to be open to such suggestions.

In one controlled study, hypnosis decreased symptoms of pain and fatigue in subjects with fibromyalgia. While more studies are needed to determine its effectiveness, hypnosis has few or no side effects.

Hypnotists aren't required to be licensed, so it's important to use caution when seeking a professional. Consult your doctor to find a reputable practitioner. Many licensed psychotherapists can perform hypnosis. Using a hypnotist isn't required, however. Many people learn to hypnotize themselves with the help of books and tapes.

GUIDED IMAGERY

Guided imagery, also called *visualization,* is a technique where the person with fibromyalgia imagines herself or himself in a pleasant situation as a way to promote relaxation or pain relief. Practitioners may act as a "guide" for the person, leading him through relaxation exercises and then to imagining certain placid scenarios (walking through a forest, swimming in the ocean). Another image is that the person's pain is water flowing down a drain and out of his body. Guided imagery may be taught in a group or private therapy session (such as by a psychotherapist or other mental-health professional) or practiced by the person on his own.

There has been little research conducted to determine the effectiveness of guided imagery in relieving pain or fatigue symp-

Evaluating Alternative and Complementary Therapies

When you're considering a complementary therapy, be cautious. In your search for relief you may be willing to try something that holds little promise. In addition to the treatments that may help, some may hurt you. Some therapies are promoted by people with little concern for your well-being, people who want only to make money.

BE PARTICULARLY SKEPTICAL OF THERAPIES THAT:

- claim to work by a secret formula

- say they are a cure or a miraculous breakthrough

- are publicized in the backs of magazines, over the phone or through direct mail (bona fide treatments will be reported in medical journals)

- rely only on testimonials as proof that they work

IN ADDITION, AS YOU ARE CONSIDERING AN ALTERNATIVE OR COMPLEMENTARY THERAPY, KEEP THE FOLLOWING ADVICE IN MIND:

Most of these therapies are not regulated. Although drugs and other conventional therapies are monitored and regulated by government agencies like the FDA, therapies such as herbs, supplements and some other alternative treatments do not have to undergo that type of scrutiny. They are not subject to approval by the FDA. So before you try an alternative treatment, learn as much as you can about it. A good source of information is the National Institute of Health's National Center for Complementary and Alternative Medicine (NCCAM). For a free packet of information on alternative therapies, write to the NCCAM Clearinghouse, P.O. Box 8218, Silver Spring, MD 20807-8218.

Discuss the therapy with your doctor. Your doctor should be informed about any therapy you're trying, whether it is an alternative remedy or an exercise program. He or she can help you watch for and safeguard against side effects and possible negative interactions with other medications you may be taking.

If you proceed, do so with caution. Seek out a qualified practitioner. Practitioners of certain therapies are required to be licensed by a state or national board. If that your state doesn't require licensing, find out about professional societies that provide certification.

Consider the cost. Some alternative therapies can be costly, and they may not be covered by your insurance. Be sure to read your policy closely to find out how much may be covered and under what circumstances.

Use good judgment. If the practitioner makes unrealistic claims (such as the therapy is a cure) or suggests that you discontinue your conventional treatments, consider it a strong warning that something is wrong.

(Adapted from: *Kids Get Arthritis Too* Newsletter, May/June 1999) toms. However, guided imagery may be a good tool for relaxation, thereby reducing anxiety and stress. Guided imagery may help relax muscles, alleviating some pain. There are no side effects. Consult your physician to discuss the addition of guided imagery to your traditional treatment program.

Remedies From Nature: Herbs and Supplements

If you've seen any magazine or television ads lately, then you know that herbs and herbal supplements are a booming business these days. Herbal remedies are increasingly available to consumers who want help for everything from depression to weight loss and even chronic illnesses like arthritis. And people are buying and using them in record numbers. A recent study by the Hartman Group revealed that sales of vitamins, minerals, herbs and other dietary supplements are around $10.4 billion a year.

Herbs and supplements are appealing to people with chronic conditions like fibromyalgia. People with fibromyalgia often are frustrated by the seeming lack of relief traditional medicine provides. They may hope that so-called natural remedies will offer a gentler type of relief for their pain with fewer unwelcome side effects. This may not always be the case.

Supplements offer the convenience of popping a pill or potion along with the idea that the organic ingredients pose little danger. But *natural* doesn't always mean *safe*. Some people think that supplements – especially herbs –

are safer than the synthetic chemicals used in over-the-counter or prescription drugs. But herbs are chemicals, too. Remember, anything with the potential to help can also be strong enough to hurt.

Because of the increased use and interest in herbs and other supplements, researchers are beginning to investigate the effects and safety of these compounds to determine if the claims are valid and if these products have a potential role in treating fibromyalgia. For most herbs and supplements, there just isn't enough scientific evidence to draw a conclusion about their efficacy. These remedies are not required to undergo the same safety and effectiveness testing that pharmaceutical drugs do because they are not regulated by the FDA. It can be difficult to tell what you are getting.

If you decide to try supplements, take care when choosing a product. Here are some other tips to help you:

• Choose products sold by large, well-established manufacturers that can be held accountable for their products.

• Ask your doctor and pharmacist what they recommend.

• Read the label to make sure the ingredient list makes sense to you. Ask your pharmacist for help if you have trouble.

• Choose products that say "standardized" on the label. Also look for "USP" on the label, which means the manufacturer has followed the U.S. Pharmacopeia's standards.

• Take note of any side effects you experience and notify your doctor.

• Consult your doctor before trying any herbal remedy or other supplement. And don't stop your current prescribed treatment.

Here's a rundown of therapies that may have some beneficial effects for fibromyalgia.

SAM-E

Also called S-adenosylmethionine, SAM-e is a naturally occurring substance that may relieve pain as well as NSAIDs do without those drugs' stomach-related side effects. Several studies also have found that SAM-e helps ease depression, leading some doctors to believe it may benefit people with fibromyalgia. However, research on SAM-e's effectiveness has been mixed. More scientific studies are needed to determine whether or not the supplement is effective.

SAM-e is a natural compound in cells that helps the body produce and regulate hormones and other biochemical substances that affect mood. SAM-e is taken in either injection or pill form and can be an expensive treatment. Because folic acid plays a role in SAM-e production, you can increase your body's production of it by eating more green, leafy vegetables. Side effects are unusual with SAM-e, but speak to your doctor before considering taking this supplement, particularly if you suffer from severe depression.

MAGNESIUM AND MALIC ACID

Magnesium is a mineral essential to healthy bone and tissue. In supplement form, it is often used in treating heart disease and other conditions. Magnesium is found in many foods, such as nuts and whole grains. Malic acid is found in apples (its name is derived from the Latin word for apple) and other fruits.

Together these supplements are touted as offering relief from the pain and fatigue of fibromyalgia. But there have been no placebo-controlled, blind studies to prove their effectiveness yet. However, some fibromyalgia experts believe that high doses of the two in supplement form may have some benefit.

Both magnesium and malic acid are involved in more effective production of ATP, a phosphate that provides a source of energy in many metabolic processes. In other words, calories from food are converted to ATP and then are used by the body as fuel. The muscle pain common in fibromyalgia could be the result of a deficiency in ATP. Although not definitively proven to provide relief from pain or fatigue associated with fibromyalgia, taking magnesium and malic acid supplements may help, and some doctors recommend their use. Patients with kidney problems should not take these supplements. One possible side effect is loose stool, such as with the use of milk-of-magnesia laxative products.

ST. JOHN'S WORT

St. John's wort is a small, yellow wildflower found in Europe and prescribed there for depression. It has become a popular herbal supplement in the United States and is sold in most drugstores and health-food stores. St. John's wort has fewer unpleasant side effects than some medications prescribed for fibromyalgia depression, such as *Prozac*. But its effectiveness has not been fully proven by scientific studies.

Although scientists don't know exactly how St. John's wort works, it contains two chemicals, hypericin and hyperforin, which may raise levels of serotonin, the brain chemical associated with depression and often found in lower-than-normal levels in people with fibromyalgia. The flower, taken in pill or liquid form, also may function as an anti-inflammatory. St. John's wort should not be taken in conjunction with other antidepressants or for serious depression. One possible side effect is increased sensitivity to the sun, so those taking the supplement should use caution.

CHLORELLA PYRENOIDOSA

In a study of 18 people with fibromyalgia, researchers at the Medical College of Virginia in Richmond found that chlorella, an alga, may help relieve fibromyalgia pain when taken in supplement form. After two months on the supplement, seven out of 18 participants in a study felt improvement in their symptoms. However, most patients also developed diarrhea and abdominal cramping. Still, the findings were promising enough to warrant a larger clinical study.

ILL-ADVISED TREATMENTS

A number of supplements and other remedies purported to relieve fibromyalgia symptoms have not been proven effective; yet unfounded, unscientific claims about these remedies continue to circulate. Consult your physician before taking any of the following supplements, and be wary of any unscientific claims concerning their supposed effectiveness.

- **Guaifenesin** is an ingredient in many cough syrups and decongestants that some people claim reduces or even banishes their fibromyalgia symptoms by increasing the excretion of *uric acid*, or phosphate, from the body. Some proponents believe that phosphate depletes energy. However, no studies have confirmed this assertion. For example, in one high-quality study by Dr. Bennett at Oregon Health Sciences University, no differences were found between women with fibromyalgia who took guaifenesin and those women who took a placebo. In fact, Dr. Bennett found no evidence that guaifenesin even causes an excretion of uric acid, let alone any indication that phosphate excretion is beneficial.
- **CMO,** short for cetyl myristoleate or cerasomal-cis-9-cetylmyristoleate, is a dietary supplement made from beef fat that some people believe can cure various forms of arthritis, including fibromyalgia. But no accepted evidence backs this claim. In the early 1990s, a promising test on rats showed that CMO protected them from arthritis, but no studies on humans have been published.
- **Gin-soaked raisins** is a folk remedy that may sound tasty, but probably is ineffective for fibromyalgia or other chronic pain syndromes. Raisins have no analgesic powers,

and alcohol, although it may dull pain temporarily, also can worsen depression and rob your body of nutrients.

CHECKLIST FOR EVALUATING ALTERNATIVE REMEDIES

Use this list to judge potential treatments with a critical eye:

Is it likely to work for me? Suspect an unproven remedy if it

- uses only case histories or testimonials as proof;
- cites only one study as proof;
- cites a study without a control group (a group of people who did not receive the treatment);
- bases findings on control and treatment groups that were not similar in age, sex, disease severity and so on;
- cites results that could have been caused by something else besides the studied treatment.

How safe is the treatment? What possible dangers may it have? Suspect an unproven remedy if it

- comes without directions for proper use;
- does not list contents;
- has no information or warnings about side effects;
- is described as harmless;
- is a diet that eliminates any basic food or nutrient or stresses eating only a few foods.

How is it promoted? Suspect an unproven remedy if it

- claims it is based on a secret formula;
- claims it cures fibromyalgia;
- cites 100 percent success (no treatment for any medical condition is 100 percent successful);
- is available only from one source;
- is evaluated only in the media, in books, or in mail-order brochures, rather than in a reputable, scientific journal.

Part Two

Chapter 4

Medical Managers:

Dealing With Your Doctor

If you don't have a doctor, find one immediately. Your doctor will be the best guide to managing your fibromyalgia, your medications and the changes fibromyalgia introduces in your life. Finding the right doctor for you — in addition to other health-care professionals such as psychiatrists or physical therapists, should you need their services — is the first step in developing a successful fibromyalgia treatment plan.

Finding a Doctor

How do you find a doctor if you don't have one? Or how do you find a specialist who will have a better understanding of fibromyalgia? If you know people with fibromyalgia who are happy with their treatment, ask them for a recommendation. You can also call the Arthritis Foundation (call 800/283-7800 to find the chapter nearest you) for a referral list of arthritis specialists in your area. Don't simply choose the first name on the list. Interview a few doctors to determine their knowledge of, interest in and attitude toward fibromyalgia. (See "Searching for a Top Doc?" on page 45.)

If you have a primary-care doctor, he or she may recommend that you see a *rheumatologist,*

a doctor who specializes in treating people with fibromyalgia and rheumatic diseases. Your doctor also may refer you, depending on your symptoms, to other medical specialists such as a physical therapist, occupational therapist, nurse, patient educator or counselor.

Remember that you're looking for a partner to join your health-care team, a set of people who will manage (along with you) your fibromyalgia. A good partnership depends on trusting your doctor's knowledge and abilities, and on feeling comfortable with him or her. To discover which qualities are most important to you, think about the doctors you have visited in the past. What did you like or dislike about them? What qualities would your ideal doctor possess? Remember that no physician is ideal, but it's important to find someone you can trust and feel confident about.

Your doctor will guide you in managing the physical aspects of living with fibromyalgia, most likely recommending:

- a balance of rest and activity
- an exercise program
- medications

Join Your Health-Care Team

Managing your fibromyalgia also means taking an active role with your doctor and any other health-care professionals you see. Of course, the professionals you use will depend on your needs and the restrictions imposed by your insurance. But whether you see several doctors or one, communication needs to be two-way. This practice ensures the best fit between recommendations for treatment and your own goals. The relationship with your doctor is in some respects like a marriage partnership. Allow plenty of room for give and take, and expect disagreements as well as agreements. Both parties need to work at the relationship and show respect for each other for it to succeed.

Who's on Your Health-Care Team?

Many health professionals may be involved in your care, depending on your condition and their availability in your area. Following is a list of health-care professionals who may play a role in your treatment.

PHYSICIANS

A physician is another name for a medical doctor or osteopath. Physicians may be primary-care doctors, providing your general medical care, or they may be specialists, such as rheumatologists. Here are some physicians you may encounter as you treat and manage your fibromyalgia.

• **Rheumatologists** specialize in treating people with arthritis or related diseases that affect the joints, muscles, bones, skin and other tissues. You may be referred to a rheumatologist if you need special care or treatment. Most rheumatologists are internists (see below) who have had further training in the care of people with arthritis and related diseases. Some rheumatologists also have pediatrics training and specialize in treating children with rheumatic diseases (see p. 46).

• **Family physicians, general practitioners and primary-care physicians** provide medical care for adults and children with different types of arthritis and related conditions. They can help you find a specialist if necessary.

• **Osteopathic physicians or doctors of osteopathy** are doctors with the same level of training as medical doctors (MDs) but with a different philosophy, one that links illnesses such as fibromyalgia to malfunctions of the musculoskeletal system. Osteopaths, as they are also known, can be primary-care physicians or specialists, such as rheumatologists.

• **Internists** specialize in internal medicine and in treating adult diseases. They provide general care to adults and can help you select

Searching for a Top Doc? A Top Doctor Tells You How

Doyt L. Conn, MD, has long been acknowledged as a leader in the fields of both arthritis research and patient care. He spent 25 years on the staff of the Mayo Clinic in Rochester, Minnesota, serves as Director of Rheumatology at Emory University School of Medicine in Atlanta and holds the position of Chief of Rheumatology at Grady Health Systems in Atlanta. Here, he draws on that extensive experience to provide the following recommendations about choosing the best doctor for your care:

Don't pick a doctor from a list. Lists can tell you a doctor's specialty, and that's about all. "Many create their lists by surveying medical school department chairmen about whom they consider to be the top doctors of their medical centers," says Dr. Conn. "Often those recommendations are based on the papers the doctor publishes, the research he performs, and the presentations he makes at scientific meetings. Unfortunately, they may have little to do with the doctor's experience in treating patients."

Look for a doctor practicing in a university medical center or a large medical practice. The more interaction your doctor has had with colleagues, medical students, residents and different kinds of patients, the more able he will be, says Dr. Conn. "In a solo practice, such opportunities are limited."

Consider a doctor with experience. A young doctor fresh from medical training may be a good choice for you. But a doctor who has been in practice for many years and stays current has the advantages of knowledge and experience, says Dr. Conn. "Although my own training was important and prepared me well to begin medical practice, I believe that with experience I became a better doctor over the years."

Choose a doctor whose focus is patients, not research. A doctor who spends more time on research than seeing patients may not be the best choice, says Dr. Conn. "There's no substitute for years of one-on-one experience with patients."

Find a doctor who is a good listener. No medical school can teach a doctor how to listen, but that's also important. Listening includes allowing you to participate in treatment decisions. Says Dr. Conn, "A doctor's concern for you and his provision of the best possible care is what matters most."

specialists. Internists should not be confused with interns, who are doctors doing a year's training in a hospital after graduating from medical school.

• **Pediatricians** treat childhood diseases and can help refer you to specialists if your child has fibromyalgia.

• **Pediatric rheumatologists** are specialists who treat children and adolescents with rheumatic conditions, and they can treat youngsters with fibromyalgia.

• **Physiatrists** (pronounced *fiz-i-aa-trists*) may direct your physical therapy, working on maintaining strength and flexibility.

• **Psychiatrists** (pronounced *sy-ky-a-trists*) are medical doctors who treat mental or emotional problems that need special attention. They can prescribe medications for treating the problems whereas *psychologists* (see Other Health Professionals, below) cannot. A psychiatrist may help if you suffer from depression or anxiety resulting from your fibromyalgia. He or she also may prescribe medications such as antidepressants.

OTHER HEALTH PROFESSIONALS

Many other health professionals may offer you assistance in managing your fibromyalgia. Some may be part of your doctor's office staff. Others may be outside health professionals that your doctor can recommend. Check your insurance policy to determine if additional treatments and health-care services are covered.

• **Chiropractors,** or doctors of chiropractic, are not medical doctors, but health-care professionals who subscribe to a philosophy that disease stems from a malalignment of the spine. Chiropractors perform spinal manipulations known as *adjustments.* Chiropractors are not licensed to prescribe medications.

• **Nurses and nurse practitioners** may be trained in treating arthritis and related illnesses such as fibromyalgia and can assist your doctor with your treatment. They also help teach you about your treatment program and can answer many of your questions.

• **Occupational therapists** work on stiffness, muscle control and coordination. They can teach you how to reduce strain on your muscles while doing everyday activities. They can fit you with stress-reducing splints and other devices. They also can help you set up a more comfortable, ergonomically sound (designed to reduce joint and muscle strain) work environment.

• **Pharmacists** fill your prescriptions for medicines and can explain drugs' actions and possible side effects. Pharmacists can tell you how different medicines work together – or interact with each other – and answer questions about prescriptions, supplements and over-the-counter medicines.

• **Physical therapists** can show you exercises to keep your muscles strong and flexible, and they can work with you to calm acute flares. They also can teach you to use special equipment that will enable you to move better. Some physical therapists are trained to design individualized fitness programs for cardiovascular health maintenance and weight control.

Personally Speaking Stories from real people with fibromyalgia

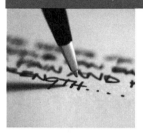

"'Seventy is the sum of our years, or eighty if we are strong.' This is a prayer that I used to chant when I was in the convent. During those 17 years when I was the good sister, I took everything we were taught to heart. We were encouraged to rise above any sickness, discomfort, fatigue or pain. For whatever these instructions were worth, this mentality is still ingrained in my mind and throughout every fiber of my being.

Living With Fibromyalgia
Mary Jucius
Arbor Vitae, WI

"I am now 56 years old, but my daily aches and fatigue sometimes make me feel as if I'm much older. I was diagnosed with fibromyalgia in March 2000. My mornings are the most difficult. I rise at about 6:30 a.m. but do not shine until about 10 a.m. Once I get moving, exercise, eat breakfast and take my meds, I feel better.

"For the past six years, I have suffered with tendinitis in both of my feet. I had major surgery, reconstruction of the post-tibia tendon, in 1997. Fibromyalgia aggravates this condition. It's a good thing I live in the woods, because I wear hiking boots with orthotics every day and everywhere I go. I am on temporary Social Security disability. However, I still need to work to survive financially. My Social Security benefits are enough to cover health insurance for my husband and me, and to help pay for my medication. I work part time for the Department of Human Resources in their Supportive Elderly Care Program. I also work at the deli at a small grocery store in town. This is hard on my muscles, but I can withstand it for four hours, twice a week.

"I like to direct my energy into creative projects. At present, I am big on rubber stamping and have enhanced my cards by learning various techniques.

"How do I cope with my fibromyalgia? I try to:

Recognize it as a chronic condition;

Respond to it by eating nutritious food;

Restore my body with vitamins and exercise;

Read inspirational and educational health books;

Respect and use my own God-given talents;

Reverence God and all of His creations, and

Rise above depression.

" I may or may not live until I'm 80 years old, but my spirit is strong and I do appreciate each day as a gift to be internalized."

Remember to "Take P.A.R.T."

Always follow these four steps to achieve success when working with your medical managers:

P – Prepare a list of questions, concerns and symptoms to discuss with your doctor.

A – Ask questions during your appointment so you understand your treatment.

R – Repeat what your doctor instructs so you can be sure you understand.

T – Take action to reduce your barriers to treatments and make the treatments more effective.

• **Physician's assistants** are trained, certified and licensed medical professionals who assist physicians by taking histories, performing physical examinations, diagnosing and treating commonly encountered medical problems under the physician's supervision. In many states, physician's assistants can prescribe medications.

• **Podiatrists,** or doctors of podiatry, specialize in foot care. They can recommend footwear that will prevent undue muscle strain in your feet and legs.

• **Psychologists** can help you solve emotional or mental problems, such as the depression that often accompanies fibromyalgia. Unlike psychiatrists, they do not have a medical degree (MD or DO) and, therefore, cannot prescribe medications. They often work in conjunction with a physician or psychiatrist.

• **Social workers** can help you find solutions to social and financial problems related to your fibromyalgia.

Prepare Before Your Visit

Fibromyalgia is a taxing condition not just for you but for members of your health-care team as well. Both health-care professionals and their patients may get frustrated from time to time when answers aren't as precise as you'd like or when treatments don't seem to be working. Doctors also can feel frustrated by too many questions that are not prioritized or that come just as a session is closing. Preparing for a visit can help minimize such frustrations. The following suggestions are some steps to take before your visit:

• Always make an appointment; don't visit the doctor's office without one. If you are having a severe flare, call your doctor's office first thing in the morning and get an appointment.

• Arrange to have your medical records transferred to the doctor's office if you are a new patient.

• Write down everything you want to ask or tell your doctor. Consider keeping a diary or journal. Write out your questions in order of priority, realizing that probably only two or three may get answered during the visit due to time constraints.

• Be prepared to describe the sequence and time when your symptoms usually begin to bother you. Use a self-monitoring form, a diary or other record sheet to keep track of your fibromyalgia symptoms between visits. Typical questions your doctor will ask include the following examples: Where are your symptoms? When did they start? Have they changed over time? How long have they lasted?

• Prepare a summary of what has happened since your last visit to the doctor. Your doctor might ask these questions: Have you been following your treatment plan? How have you been feeling? Have you had any problems? What has been happening in your life? Jot down answers to these kinds of questions ahead of time.

• When evaluating a particular treatment, give it some time before deciding if it's failed. Allow several weeks on a treatment to see if it is having a noticeable effect. Tell your doctor if you have trouble following recommendations.

• Finding the right treatment may involve trying several that don't work out. After a trial period on a new treatment, if you don't feel better, let your doctor or other health-care professional know that you need to try something else.

• Keep a log of the names and the dosages of all medicines you're taking, including prescription and over-the-counter drugs. If you're taking several medications, you may wish to bring your pill bottles with you to your appointment. This suggestion is especially important if you're visiting more than one doctor.

• If you are seeing your doctor on a return visit, make a list of any medication refills you need. Be prepared to discuss any medicines that are not helping or that are causing side effects.

• Note any alternative treatments you are using. Even though the doctor didn't prescribe the treatment, he or she should know you are taking it.

DURING THE VISIT

Handle your doctor's visit like a business appointment. Come prepared, ask for what you need, repeat what you heard, and take action to deal with any barriers that may affect your treatment plan.

Think ahead about what you would like to accomplish in your visit. Prepare to give your doctor an overview of how you have been doing since the last visit, not just the last few days or weeks.

Prepare a list of questions to ask your doctor during the visit. Cover your most important concerns first, and be concise. Patients often experience many symptoms and may try to discuss a lengthy list that cannot be addressed in a single visit. Report to the doctor the reason for your visit and what you want him or her to do today.

Tell the doctor about your symptoms, as well as changes in your life that may affect your fibromyalgia, your self-help activities, problems with treatment, results of visits to other health professionals, your current list of medications, and any other updates relevant to your treatment plan. Give honest, accurate information about your concerns, any alternative or complementary remedies you've tried or changes you have made in your treatment regimen. Your doctor can safely recommend treatments only if he or she has the full picture.

During the appointment, try to obtain any of the following information you do not already have:

• your diagnosis and how your condition affects you

• the purpose, risks and results of any tests
• the choices for treatment and the benefits, risks and side effects of each treatment
• when to call the doctor about side effects of medications or lack of response to a treatment
• how a particular treatment should be performed

It's easy to forget or misunderstand instructions. Repeat the key points you've heard during the visit, such as diagnosis, prognosis, next steps, treatment actions and so on. Repetition will allow your doctor to clarify anything that has been confusing and will help you remember what was discussed.

Take notes or ask if the doctor has any written handouts or brochures, or if he or she can give you written instructions about any prescribed treatments.

Take part in decisions about treatment by sharing your goals and preferences. Let the doctor know any possible barriers to following his or her recommendations such as financial concerns, conflicts with sleep, eating habits or daily schedule.

Keep an open mind when working with your doctor. No single treatment is best for everyone with fibromyalgia. If something does not work, let your doctor know so you can try something else. It may take a long time to find the right treatment.

DISCUSSING ALTERNATIVE THERAPIES

More Americans are trying alternative therapies, and people with fibromyalgia are no exception. One Canadian study found that 70 percent of people with fibromyalgia have tried an over-the-counter rub, 40 percent have consulted an alternative practitioner and 26 percent have tried special diets in an effort to alleviate their symptoms. If you are considering using any alternative therapy, begin by talking to your doctor. Here's how:

• Be candid about any alternative medicines you are already taking. Your doctor can't help you or protect you if he or she doesn't know the whole story.

• Tell your doctor about any therapies you are considering, and share what you have been reading or hearing about various therapies.

• Ask your doctor what he or she knows about any therapy you are considering, especially any possible dangers such as drug interactions with medications you are taking. Also ask your doctor to refer you to an established practitioner, or to write you a prescription. Both will improve your chances for insurance coverage.

• If your doctor objects to the treatments you propose, find out why. If you still want to consider the option, check with another doctor, or consider changing doctors. Although doctors are increasingly open to combining traditional and complementary medicine, not all of them favor this approach.

Use the following worksheets to prepare for your next appointment. Make copies if you need to so that you'll have them for future visits or for visits with other members of your health-care team. These can be guidelines to becoming an active participant in the treatment of your fibromyalgia.

"ASK THE DOCTOR" Worksheet

Complete this part before the visit:

1. What is the main reason I am going to the doctor?

   _____

   _____

2. Is there anything else that concerns me about my health or treatment (e.g., effect of fibromyalgia on work, family or mood; problems following the recommended treatment plan)?

   _____Yes _____No

   _____

3. What do I want the doctor to do today?

   _____

   _____

4. The symptoms that bother me the most are ... (What? Where? When did they start? Do they change over time? How long do they last?). NOTE: bring copies of any completed self-monitoring forms/diaries.

   _____

   _____

5. What medications (prescriptions and over-the-counter) am I taking regularly? (List name(s) and dosage, or take the bottles to your appointment.)

   _____

   _____

6. What are my goals for treatment (what I want or expect to get out of treatment)?

   _____

   _____

7. Prepare and prioritize a list of questions to give the doctor early in the visit.

   _____

   _____

8. Do I need Medicare, Medicaid or other insurance cards/forms today?

   _____Yes_____ No

"ASK THE DOCTOR" Worksheet

Questions to ask your doctor during the visit:

1. What is happening to me? How is my fibromyalgia likely to affect me?

   _____

2. What are the results of my tests, and what do they mean? May I have a copy of the results?

   _____

3. Why do I need the lab tests or X-rays that you are recommending today?

   _____

4. Are there any risks from these tests?

   _____

5. When should I call for the results?

   _____

6. What should I do at home (diet, activity, treatment options, special instructions, medications, precautions, etc.)?

   _____

a. What are the benefits, costs and drawbacks for each option for treatment?

   _____

b. How and how often do I do the treatment?

   _____

c. How long should I give it a try?

   _____

7. When should I call if my condition doesn't improve and the treatment doesn't seem to be working? What symptoms warrant my calling before my next scheduled visit?

   _____

8. When should I return for another visit?

   _____

"ASK THE DOCTOR" Worksheet

Medication questions:

1. What is the name of the drug? _____

2. What are the purpose and benefits of this drug?
   _____

3. How quickly does it work? How long should I take this drug?
   _____

4. What are the possible side effects or drawbacks to the drug?
   _____

   a. When should I contact you about side effects?
   _____

   b. What can I do to prevent or deal with the side effects or drawbacks?
   _____

5. Is it all right to take the drug with other drugs (such as cold, sinus, allergy, pain medicines) I am taking? _____Yes_____No
   If not, what drugs should I avoid?_____

6. When is the best time to take the drug? Before, with or after meals?
   _____

7. What should I do if I forget to take my medicine?
   _____

8. Are there any changes I should make in my diet? _____Yes _____No
   If so, what?_____

   a. Can I drink alcohol while taking this drug? _____Yes _____No

   b. Are there any other restrictions?_____Yes _____No
   If so, what? _____

9. Should I avoid driving while taking this drug? _____Yes _____ No

10. Is a generic drug available? If so, is generic as effective? _____ Yes _____ No

Part Three

Develop a
Good Living Lifestyle

Chapter 5

Managing Your Lifestyle:

Elements of Good Living

Doctors increasingly agree that many factors influence chronic illness and the way it affects us. Illness does not occur in a vacuum. How we approach the other parts of our lives, our attitudes, our expectations, our sense of control and general well-being all affect how we feel, whether we have a chronic illness or not. It's true that you cannot change the fact that you have fibromyalgia. But you can control how well you take care of yourself, both mentally and physically. Finding a healthy balance between exercise and rest, eating a nutritious diet and nourishing your mind and spirit inevitably will affect how you feel.

The Keys to Good Living

Good living with fibromyalgia means working hard to lead a healthy life, and much of that you can accomplish through improving your attitude and outlook. In important ways, fibromyalgia is a syndrome that requires placing mind over matter. The following sections offer some techniques for improving your outlook and achieving good living.

OPTIMISM

Over the past decade, researchers increasingly have confirmed the connection between the mind and the body. Working to control and enjoy your life can reduce your level of chronic stress and even help you live longer. But positive attitudes take some work, such as setting realistic goals. Write down each problem you associate with fibromyalgia and the ways you can tackle it. Avoid doing things you dislike, and cultivate friendships with people whose outlook you admire. Try some new activities, and cut back on the ones that tire or depress you. Counter pessimistic thoughts with realistic judgments. For example, your new medication may help reduce your pain, and the exercise program may increase your strength and energy. You'll have to be persistent about positive thinking, but the results are worth the effort.

HUMOR

Laughter really is good medicine. Author Norman Cousins refers to laughing as "internal jogging." Anything that makes you smile brings relief to your mind and spirit. Some research has shown that humor may even improve your immune system functions. (See Chapter 10 for more on humor.)

SENSE OF PURPOSE

Do you believe that you have worth and a purpose for your life and experiences? People who believe in themselves and in the meaning of their lives are happier, more satisfied and serene. This belief in one's self is a choice that occurs regardless of life circumstances.

SENSE OF CONTROL

Do you feel helpless or continually frustrated by your fibromyalgia or other challenges in your life? Given the same situation, some people will choose to feel helpless. Others will feel a sense of control, a confidence that they can help influence their own well-being. Goal-setting and contracting, problem-solving, self-monitoring, keeping a journal, communicating with others about your needs and planning are all ways to regain a sense of control.

SOCIAL SUPPORT

Is your life filled with satisfying relationships and love? Do you feel that others understand your fibromyalgia and the demands that it places on you? Are you getting the support that you need? Getting that support can be hard work, but this issue is important for many people with fibromyalgia. Many people with fibromyalgia struggle to explain their illness and their particular needs to family, friends, bosses and co-workers. You need to be a friend to have a friend, and you need to be willing to listen to others as well as communicate your own needs in a clear, direct way.

POSITIVE SELF-IMAGE

The way you feel about yourself is an important part of good living. Chronic pain and fatigue can drag you down and make you feel as if there's no point in taking care of yourself. Counteract negative feelings by treating yourself better. Begin by trying the worksheet, "The Best of Me," on page 63. Objectively evaluating yourself may help you remember why you're worth pampering. Then consider some of the following ways to treat yourself:

- Get your hair cut in a new style.
- Rent a spirit-lifting video, like an action movie or a comedy.
- Spring for a pedicure or a manicure.
- Get a massage to lift your spirits and help alleviate pain.
- Start a book club. It's an easy way to socialize, without the usual labor involved in entertaining.
- Rejuvenate in a long, hot bath.
- Adopt a pet from the local animal shelter. Helping an animal can bring joy and companionship to your life.
- Pray or meditate.

Personally Speaking   Stories from real people with fibromyalgia

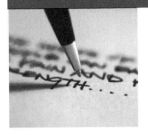

The Lessons of Fibromyalgia
Carol Reiker
Peoria, IL

"Fibromyalgia has been both a blessing and a misfortune for me. It has forced me to slow down. I now understand that I am worthy because of who I am, not what I produce. I can appreciate and enjoy the little things in life. I have learned compassion. And I have given up the control that was so much a part of my nature. God has a total plan in my life.

"The hardest part of having fibromyalgia is learning to say no. But saying no without giving a reason is also one of the most liberating things I've learned. Today, I have enough self-respect not to seek validation from other people.

"Thanks to the support of my family, I have never felt like giving up. At times, I'll see someone mowing the grass and have the sinking feeling, 'I wish I could do that.' But immediately I counteract that negativity with a positive thought.

"I can't waste my energy on self-pity. It's simply too precious."

My favorite coping tips:

- Use a heated mattress pad set on high in the morning before getting out of bed. Do slow stretches in bed while your muscles warm up. Flex your ankles and legs and roll your head from side to side.
- Before going to bed, make a list of things to do for the next day to help you organize, prioritize and relax.
- For big projects, like yard work, use the buddy system. Ask a friend or family member to do the more physically exerting tasks, such as digging holes, while you stick to manageable jobs like fertilizing or planting flowers in the holes. Use a time-released fertilizer that acts through the summer and fall so you have to do it only once.
- When entertaining, plan a menu with food that can be prepared ahead of time. Shop for groceries several days before the event. Cook moderate amounts over a period of days and freeze. Set the table well in advance. All this planning leaves you fresh and relaxed for the party.
- Double your recipes when you cook. Freeze the second batch for a later date. Also, get your family to help. Set aside two whole days for cooking, and make food for the whole month.
- Help others. It may have a positive influence on how you feel.

• Help someone else by doing a favor for a friend or through volunteer work.

• Your use of time and your balance of activities can affect your health and satisfaction. Using the Time Target on the next page, evaluate the time you spend on key activities like hobbies, time alone or with friends, family time and so on.

• Follow the instructions on the Time Target. After you have completed the worksheet, look for any patterns. Is your life balanced so that most or all of the bull's-eye (the center circle) is colored in? Or do you have many parts of the other circles colored in? Look for colored areas in the outer circles.

After completing the Time Target exercise, try completing the worksheets on the following pages to help you learn to balance your activities and feel better about yourself.

Activity: Targeting Your Time

Instructions: Read the names for each of the 12 activities listed in the wedges of the circle below. Think about how satisfied you are with the time you now spend on each activity. Color in the part of the wedge for each activity that best describes how that activity fits into your life. For example, if you are satisfied with time spent on an activity, color the center part of the wedge, in the "OK" section. Otherwise, indicate by coloring whether you "need less" or "need more" of the activity, or if the activity is "not important" in your life.

HOW CLOSE ARE YOU TO THE BULL'S-EYE?

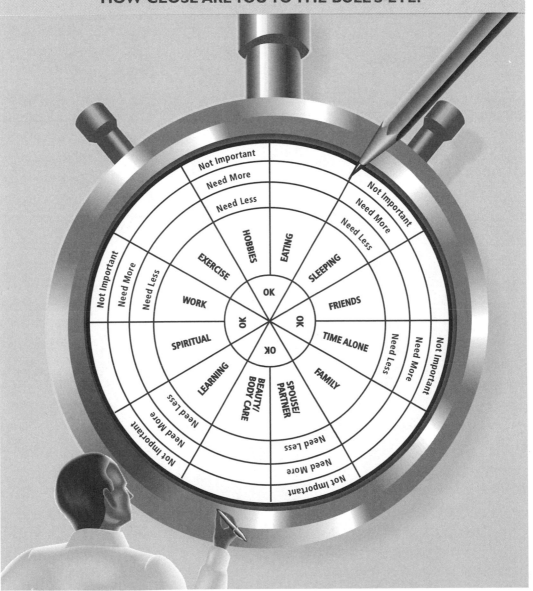

WORKSHEET: Things You Love To Do

Write down as many activities as possible that bring you enjoyment and happiness. In the "Rank Top Five" column, indicate by number those five activities that you enjoy the most. In the "Last Time" column, indicate how long it has been since you engaged in each of your top five activities.

	Activities	Rank Top Five	Last Time
1			
2			
3			
4			
5			
6			
7			
8			
9			
10			
11			
12			
13			
14			
15			

WORKSHEET: The Best of Me

List at least 10 qualities or aspects that make you unique, that you like or admire about yourself and/or that make you attractive (include at least one or two physical attributes).

1	
2	
3	
4	
5	
6	
7	
8	
9	
10	

Chapter 6

Get Moving:

The Benefits of Exercise

Why exercise? Exercise because you can't afford not to exercise. Exercise because you are tired of pain. Exercise because you want to have more control over how you feel. The best thing you can do for you and for your fibromyalgia is to exercise.

Don't let the word *exercise* throw you. Done right, exercise can be another word for recreation. It's a walk in the park, a stroll around your yard. It's something to start slowly and carefully at a pace you enjoy and are comfortable with.

Exercise Has Many Benefits

There are sound scientific reasons to exercise as well. Two principles of treatment for fibromyalgia are to increase cardiovascular (aerobic) fitness, and to stretch, mobilize and strengthen tight, sore muscles. Research has shown that exercise can improve general health and fitness without increasing fibromyalgia symptoms. In fact, regular exercise can
- keep your body from becoming too stiff;
- keep your muscles strong;
- keep bone and cartilage tissue strong and healthy;
- improve your ability to do daily activities;
- give you more energy;
- help you sleep better;

- control your weight;
- improve your cardiovascular health;
- provide an outlet for stress and tension;
- decrease depression and anxiety;
- release endorphins, your body's natural pain relievers; and
- improve your self-esteem, and provide a sense of well-being.

Still, if the idea of starting an exercise program intimidates you – and that wouldn't be surprising for anyone who suffers chronic pain – try to remind yourself how much exercise can help. The point is to start slowly and gradually increase your workout as you become stronger and increase your endurance.

(See the sample start-up program for those with fibromyalgia later in this chapter.) Don't expect to regain immediately the level of fitness you enjoyed prior to having fibromyalgia. It takes time to build up your strength and endurance. Have reasonable expectations. Just getting started is an accomplishment. Making exercise a habit is a great accomplishment.

What If I Don't Exercise?

It's natural for people in pain to guard aching body parts and reduce their activities. But going without exercise can result in a cycle of deconditioning, creating stiffness and increased muscle tension that leads to further pain, as the diagram here illustrates. Add the effects of a poor night's sleep, and who has the energy to move?

Unfortunately, the saying "use it or lose it" is true. Studies show that healthy people who are given bed rest rapidly decondition, suffer-

ing reduced cardiac output, reduced blood volume, atrophied muscles, decreased bone density and light-headedness when they get out of bed. The same is true of general inactivity. Your muscles become smaller and weaker and are less able to support and protect you. You have less stamina and tire more easily. Daily activities become more difficult. This loss in function and independence can lead to depression, anger and lowered self-esteem. These effects in turn result in stress, which creates muscle tension, leading to more pain and so on.

The good news is that exercise can break this cycle. In 1999, Canadian researchers studied 41 fibromyalgia patients and found that those who participated in a six-week exercise and educational program showed significant improvement in the distance they could walk and in their well-being, fatigue and pain. The results were immediate and sustained. Another

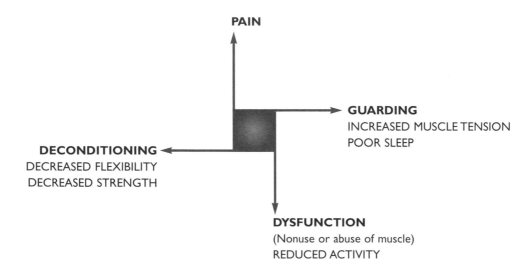

A Vicious Cycle: Pain, Guarding, Dysfunction and Deconditioning

Personally Speaking Stories from real people with fibromyalgia

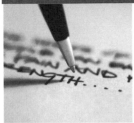

"**H**iking, biking and walking several miles each day used to be a cinch for me. But when fibromyalgia moved into my legs, I could barely make it from my car to my office.

"As I tried exercise alternatives – tai chi, a treadmill and an exercise bike – my knees screamed 'halt!' So I asked the volunteers at my Arthritis Foundation chapter what to try next. 'Try the warm-water Arthritis Foundation/YMCA aquatics program,' they suggested. 'The pool is right down the block, the water feels great, and you don't have to get your hair wet. All you need is your doctor's permission.'

Poetry In Motion
Jean Maguire
Arthritis Foundation
Rocky Mountain Chapter

"My doctor was eager to try something new. He recommended aquatics; I'd be his test case for people with fibromyalgia. He cautioned me to go slow and take it easy.

Going slow was not a problem for me. Just getting from the parking lot to the dressing room, showers and to the pool wore me out. Arriving at the pool, I gazed out at all the silver-haired people in their 70s and 80s and thought, "Great. Maybe I can keep up with them." Not so, and they were twice my age. The first month I stayed for only 10 minutes, twice per week.

"But what a glorious 10 minutes, floating free of gravity and the limits of pain. In the warm water, it felt wonderful to be able to move again, and I could move easily. My instructors were patient and encouraged me to go at my own slower pace. As I began to meet the others in the class, they added their encouragement. 'Looking better today! Keep up the good work. It takes a while. Stay with it and you'll see an improvement.'

"A few months later I was able to stay for all of the leg exercises and most of the arm exercises. In the pool, I was making good friends as we laughed, told jokes and shared stories. Outside the pool, I had more energy, better sleep and decreased pain. Going to movies and plays, or visiting friends and family were options for me again.

"After a year in the aquatics program, I strapped on a flotation belt and glided to the pool end and back. The class cheered. 'Poetry in motion,' said an 85-year-old gent. I knew I had arrived at more than the end of the pool. Being able to get my body to do what I wanted made me feel whole and beautiful again.

"Several years later, aquatics is a regular, wouldn't-miss-it, two-times-a-week part of my self-help routine. We sing 'Take Me Out to the Ball Game' in the pool, and I dreamed of actually being able to walk into a real Colorado Rockies baseball game. Thanks to aquatics, and the use of a cane and elevator, I was able to see eight games last season. Now as I cheer for the Rockies' moves, I have some great ones of my own."

study at the University of Missouri School of Medicine in Columbia found that exercise training lessened pain at tender points and improved physical functioning. Exercise was especially effective in combination with biofeedback and relaxation training.

Exercising With Chronic Pain

Exercise will help your pain, but that does not mean the exercise itself will be pain-free, especially at first. You may experience some cramping or fatigue in your muscles as you start. New pain that comes from new conditioning hurts but is not harmful. Following are some tips for exercising even when you suffer chronic pain.

• If a form of exercise, such as walking, causes you increased pain that lasts two hours after you finish, slow down next time, or decrease the duration of your workout. If those adjustments don't help, talk to your doctor.

• If you are unable to do any exercise without significant pain, talk to your doctor about a different form of exercise.

• Apply no more than 20 minutes of heat to painful areas before exercise and ten to 15 minutes of cold following your exercise. Heat increases your blood flow, which can reduce stiffness, calm excited nerve endings and relax aching muscles. Try heating pads, warm showers, baths or whirlpools before an exercise routine. Cold helps control pain and reduce muscle spasms. Use ice, cold packs or bags of frozen vegetables, such as peas, following your workout when you need relief.

• Massage stiff or sore muscles before exercising. Massage will stimulate tissues and muscles.

• Wear elastic supports for elbows, ankles and knees. These are available at drugstores or medical supply stores. Ask your doctor or physical therapist if this type of supportive device would help you.

• Use a walking stick or cane on your least affected side for stability and support. The handle should reach your wrist when your hand is by your side.

• Distract yourself while you exercise. Wear a radio headset, or exercise with a talkative friend. Think about things you look forward to, sing, recite poetry or practice a speech. Just keep your mind occupied with something else besides pain.

• Think of your pain as something else: a hot sensation, a momentary discomfort. Remind yourself that as your muscles relax into the exercise, some of the unpleasant feelings will lessen.

Talk to yourself about why you *are* exercising instead of why you *can't* exercise. Remind yourself what research shows: exercise can help. List the things exercise is accomplishing for you: strengthening your muscles, increasing your stamina, improving your mood and getting you out into the fresh air.

Three Essentials of an Exercise Program

Everyone, including people with fibromyalgia, benefits from a balanced exercise program with different types of exercise: warm-up, strengthening and endurance, and cooldown exercises.

- **Warm-up exercises.** Warm up with some easy marching, walking or arm swings before exercising. Your warm up can include range-of-motion, stretching and some strengthening exercises. Warm-up exercises safely prepare your heart and lungs for endurance and help maintain or increase flexibility and muscle strength. For some people with severe physical limitations, warm-up exercises may be the only type of exercise they can do at first.

- **Endurance exercises.** Endurance, or aerobic, exercises use the large muscles of the body and increase the heart rate. They are important for cardiovascular fitness, weight control and reducing fatigue. They include swimming, walking, bicycling and even raking leaves. Work into these activities gradually. Try thinking of aerobic exercise as a medication that raises your body's natural painkillers. Moderate doses daily are more effective than a very high dose a few times a week.

- **Cool-down exercises.** As you gradually lengthen your exercise duration, build in a cool-down period to let your body lose some of the heat generated while exercising. This cool-down will help relax your body, return your heart rate to normal and avoid sore muscles. To cool down, do your chosen aerobic exercise in slow motion for three to five minutes, followed by a few flexibility and stretching exercises.

Different Types of Exercise

To create your fitness program, you should combine some type of flexibility and muscle-strengthening exercises with endurance exercises.

You may not be able to do all of these every day. Let the way you're feeling be your guide.

RANGE-OF-MOTION (FLEXIBILITY/STRETCHING) EXERCISES

Range-of-motion exercises reduce stiffness and help keep muscles and joints flexible. The *range of motion* is the range that your joints can move comfortably in certain directions. A physical therapist can teach you appropriate range-of-motion exercises, also called flexibility or stretching exercises.

Try to move your joints through their range of motion every day. Daily activities such as housework, climbing stairs, dressing, bathing, cooking, lifting or bending do not dependably do that and should not replace range-of-motion exercises prescribed by your doctor or therapist.

You can use some range-of-motion exercises to stretch or elongate the ligaments and muscles around the joint. This stretching helps maintain or improve the flexibility of these tissues. Stretching also reduces muscle tension. A sustained, gentle, non-painful stretch to a tight muscle will assist in relaxing that muscle, improving flexibility and reducing pain.

STRENGTHENING EXERCISES

These exercises help maintain or increase muscle strength. Strong muscles keep your body conditioned and better able to withstand the painful effects of fibromyalgia. They also will help you better handle your day-to-day tasks, such as climbing stairs, carrying groceries or gardening. Two common strengthening exercises are isometric and isotonic exercises:

• **Isometric Exercises.** In these exercises, you tighten your muscles but don't move your joints. Isometrics help build the muscles around your joints. Examples include quadriceps sets, in which you tighten the large muscle on the front of your thigh muscles, and gluteal sets, in which you tighten the muscles in your buttocks. Tightening and then holding the muscle may cause rebound contractions, since you are asking a muscle to relax that doesn't know how. Instead, try tightening your muscles and immediately releasing.

• **Isotonic Exercises.** In these exercises, you move your joints to strengthen your muscles. For example, straightening your knee while sitting in a chair is an isotonic exercise that

Sample Exercises

Here are some sample range-of-motion and strengthening exercises that you can use in either a warm-up or a cool-down. Select the exercises that are best for you, avoiding those that stress already painful areas. These exercises have been excerpted from the Arthritis Foundation's PACE (People with Arthritis Can Exercise). To purchase copies of the PACE videos, call 800-207-8633 or shop online at www.arthritis.org.

NECK EXERCISES

Purpose: Increase neck movement; relax neck and shoulder muscles; improve posture.

Precautions: Do these exercises slowly and smoothly. If you feel dizzy, stop the exercise. If you have had neck problems, check with your doctor before doing these exercises.

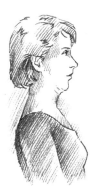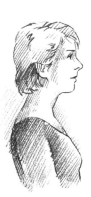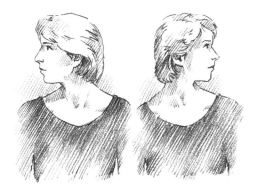

1. CHIN TUCKS	2. HEAD TURNS (ROTATION)
Pull your chin back as if to make a double chin. Keep your head straight – don't look down. Hold three seconds. Then raise your neck straight up as if someone was pulling straight up on your hair.	Turn your head to look over your shoulder. Hold three seconds. Return to the center and then turn to look over your other shoulder. Hold three seconds. Repeat.

helps strengthen your thigh muscle. Isotonic exercises include range-of-motion exercises, but they become strengthening exercises when you increase the speed or repetition of exercises, or add weight to the exercise (initially one to two pounds).

Water exercises can help strengthen muscles by increasing resistance as well as assistance to movements. Changing the position in which you do exercises also can help strengthen muscles. For example, you encounter more resistance when you raise your arms from a sitting position than when you raise your arms from a lying-down position.

Strengthening exercises must be carefully designed for people with fibromyalgia. Knowing which muscle needs to be strengthened and how to perform the exercise with-

---

SHOULDER EXERCISES

Purpose: Increase mobility of the shoulder girdle (the bony structure that supports your upper limbs); strengthen muscles that raise shoulders; relax neck and shoulder muscles.

Precautions: If the exercise increases pain, stop and consult with your physician.

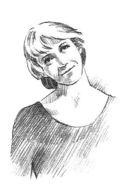 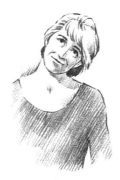 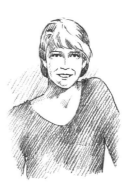 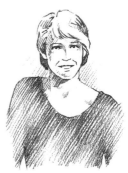

3. HEAD TILTS

Focus on an object in front of you. Tilt your head sideways toward your right shoulder. Hold three seconds. Return to the center, and tilt toward your left shoulder. Hold three seconds. Do not twist head but continue to look forward. Do not raise your shoulder toward your ear.

4. SHOULDER SHRUGS (ELEVATION)

(A) Raise one shoulder, lower it. Then raise the other shoulder; Be sure the first shoulder is completely relaxed and lowered before raising the other.
(B) Raise both shoulders up toward the ears. Hold three seconds. Relax. Concentrate on completely relaxing shoulders as they come down. Do not tilt the head or body in either direction. Do not hunch your shoulders forward or pinch shoulder blades together.

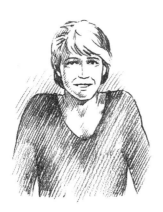
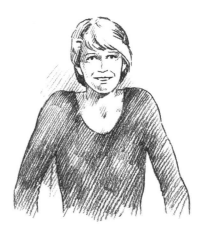

5. SHOULDER CIRCLES

Lift both shoulders up; move them forward, then down and back in a circling motion.
Then lift both shoulders up; move them backward, then down and forward in a circling motion.

ARM EXERCISES (Shoulders and Elbows)

Purpose: Increase shoulder and/or elbow motion; strengthen shoulder and/or elbow muscles; relax neck and shoulder muscles; improve posture.

Precautions: If you have had shoulder or elbow surgery, check with your surgeon before doing these exercises. These exercises are not advised for people with significant shoulder joint damage, such as unstable joints or total cuff tears.

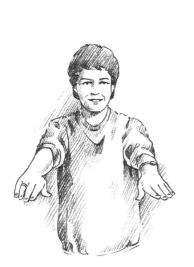
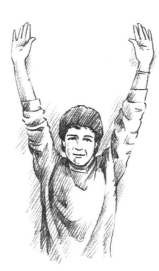

6. FORWARD ARM REACH

Raise one or both arms forward and upward as high as possible. Return to your starting position.

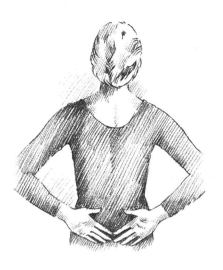

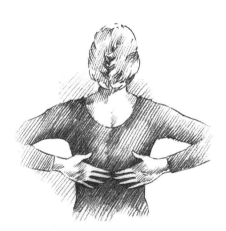

7. SELF BACK RUB (INTERNAL ROTATION)

While seated, slide a few inches forward from the back of your chair. Sit up as straight as possible; do not round your shoulders. Place the back of your hands on your lower back. Slowly move them upward until you feel a stretch in your shoulders. Hold three seconds, then slide your hands back down. You can use one hand to help the other. Move within the limits of your pain. Do not force.

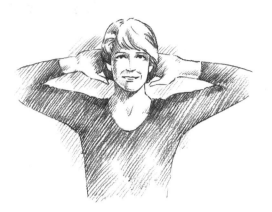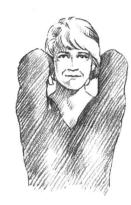

8. SHOULDER ROTATOR

Sit or stand as straight as possible. Reach up and place your hands on the back of your head. (If you cannot reach your head, place your arms in a "muscle man" position with elbows bent in a right angle and upper arm at shoulder level.) Take a deep breath in. As you breathe out, bring your elbows together in front of you. Slowly move elbows apart as you breathe in.

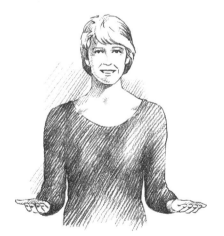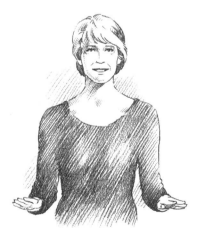

9. DOOR OPENER

Bend your elbows and hold them in to your sides. Your forearms should be parallel to the floor. Slowly turn forearms and palms to face the ceiling. Hold three seconds and then turn palms slowly toward the floor.

WRIST EXERCISES

Purpose: Increase wrist motion; strengthen wrist muscles.

Precautions: If you have had wrist or elbow surgery, check with your doctor before doing this exercise. Stop if you feel any numbness or tingling.

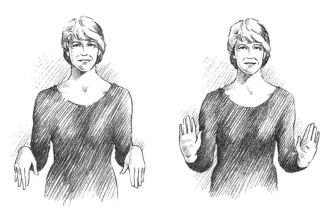

10. WRIST BEND (EXTENSION)

If sitting, rest hands and forearms on thighs, table, or arms of chair. If standing, bend your elbows and hold hands in front of you, palms down. Lift palms and fingers, keeping forearms flat. Hold three seconds. Relax.

FINGER EXERCISES

Purpose: Increase finger motion; increase ability to grip and hold objects.

Precautions: If the exercise increases finger pain, stop and consult with your doctor.

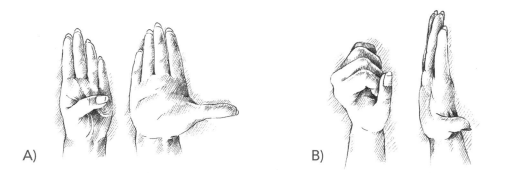

A)

B)

11. THUMB BEND AND FINGER CURL (FLEXION/EXTENSION)

(A) With hands open and fingers relaxed, reach thumb across your palm and try to touch the base of your little finger. Hold three seconds. Stretch thumb back out to the other side as far as possible. (B) Make a loose fist by curling all your fingers into your palm. Keep your thumb out. Hold for three seconds. Then stretch your fingers to straighten them.

TRUNK EXERCISES

Purpose: Increase trunk flexibility; stretch and strengthen back and abdominal muscles.

Precautions: If you have osteoporosis or have had back compression fracture, previous back surgery or a hip replacement, check with your doctor before doing these exercises. Do not bend your body forward or backward unless specifically told to do so. Move slowly and immediately stop any exercise that causes you back or neck pain.

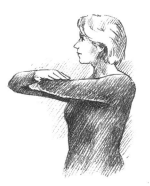

12. SIDE BENDS
While standing, keep weight evenly on both hips with knees slightly bent. Lean toward the right and reach your fingers toward the floor. Hold three seconds. Return to center and repeat exercise toward the left. Do not lean forward or backward while bending, and do not twist the torso.

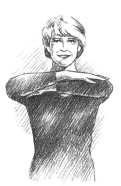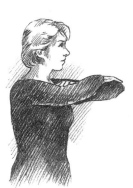

13. TRUNK TWIST (ROTATION)
Place your hands on your hips, straight out to the side, crossed over your chest, or on opposite elbows. Twist your body around to look over your right shoulder. Hold three seconds. Return to the center and then twist to the left. Be sure you are twisting at the waist and not at your neck or hips. NOTE: Vary the exercise by holding a ball in front of or next to your body.

LOWER-BODY EXERCISES

Purpose: Increase lower-body strength; increase range of motion in hip, knee and ankle joints.

Precautions: Check with your surgeon before doing these exercises if you have had hip, knee, ankle, foot or toe surgery, or any lower-extremity joint replacement. Do not rotate the upper body unless specifically told to do so. When standing, bend your knees slightly to avoid "locking" your knee joints.

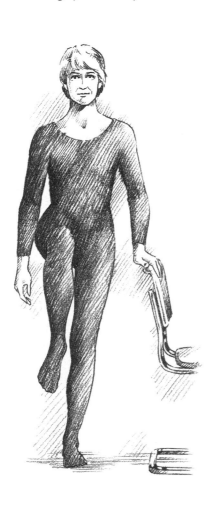

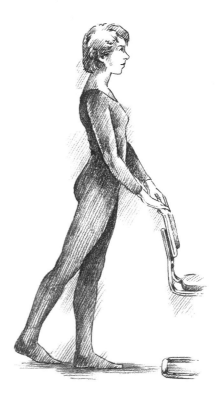

15. BACK KICK (HIP EXTENSION)

Stand straight on one leg and lift the other leg behind you. Hold three seconds. Try to keep your leg straight as you move it backward. Motion should occur only in the hip (not the waist). Do not lean forward – keep your upper body straight. NOTE: You can add resistance by using a large rubber exercise band around ankles.

14. MARCH (HIP/KNEE FLEXION)

Stand sideways to a chair and lightly grasp the back. If you feel unsteady, hold onto two chairs or face the back of the chair. Alternate lifting your legs up and down as if marching in place. Gradually try to lift knees higher and/or march faster.

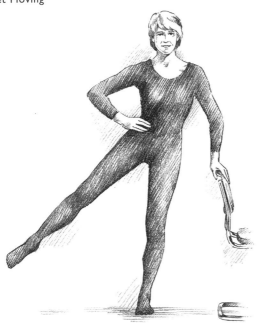

16. SIDE LEG KICK (HIP ABDUCTION/ADDUCTION)

Stand near a chair, holding it for support. Stand on one leg and lift the other leg out to the side. Hold three seconds and return your leg to the floor. Only move your leg at the top – don't lean toward the chair. Alternate legs.

Precautions: Check with your surgeon before doing these exercises if you have had a hip replacement. Keep the knee bent in the weight-bearing leg. Don't rotate your upper body – keep your chest and shoulders facing forward.

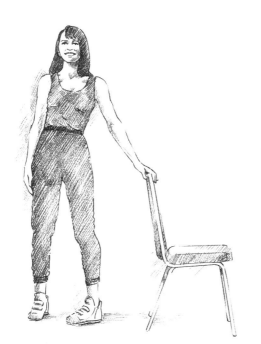

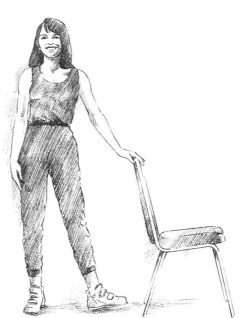

17. HIP TURNS (HIP INTERNAL/EXTERNAL ROTATION)

Stand with legs slightly apart, with your weight on one leg and the heel of your other foot lightly touching the floor. Rotate your whole leg from the hip so that toes and knee point in and then out. Don't rotate your body – keep chest and shoulders facing forward. NOTE: If you have difficulty putting weight on one leg, you can do this exercise by sitting at the edge of a chair with your legs extended straight in front and your heels resting on the floor.

Precautions: Check with your surgeon before doing these exercises if you have had a hip replacement. Don't rotate your upper body – keep your chest and shoulders facing forward.

Precautions: Do not do the following exercise if you have had ankle or foot surgery. Stop if you experience calf pain or cramping.

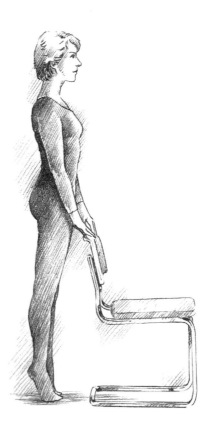

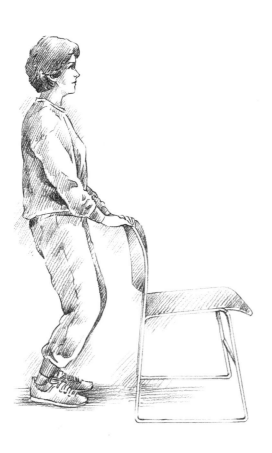

18. SKIER'S SQUAT (QUADRICEPS STRENGTHENER)

Stand behind a chair with your hands lightly resting on top of the chair for support. Keep your feet flat on the floor. Keeping your back straight, slowly bend your knees to lower your body a few inches. Hold for three to six seconds, then slowly return to an upright position.

19. TIPTOE (DORSI/PLANTAR FLEXION)

Face the back of a chair and rest your hands on it. Rise and stand on your toes. Hold three seconds, then return to the flat position. Try to keep your knees straight (but not locked). Now stand on your heels, raising your toes and front part of your foot off the ground. NOTE: You can do this exercise one foot at a time.

Precautions: If you have had recent ankle surgery, check with your surgeon before doing the following exercise.

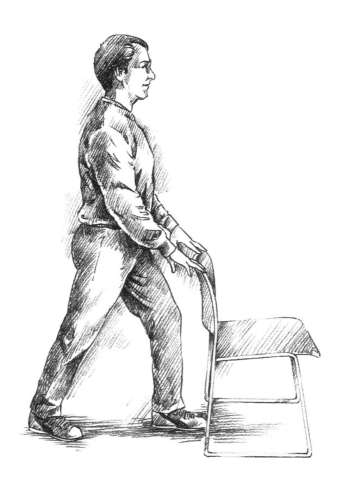

20. CALF STRETCH (GASTROC-SOLEUS STRETCH)

Hold lightly to the back of a chair. Bend the knee of the leg you are not stretching so that it almost touches the chair. Put the leg to be stretched behind you, keeping both feet flat on the floor. Lean forward gently, keeping your back knee straight.

Precautions: Stop if the following exercises increase your back pain.

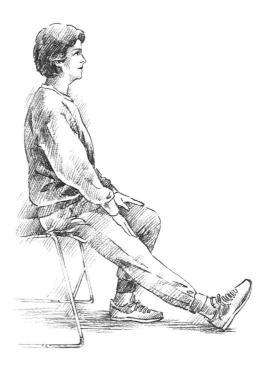

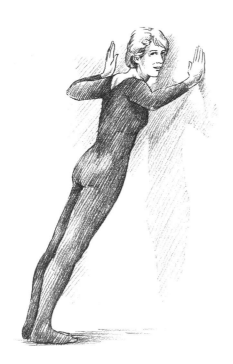

21. CHEST STRETCH (HIP EXTENSION AND PECTORALIS STRETCH)

Stand about two to three feet away from a wall and place your hands or forearms on the wall at shoulder height. Lean forward, leading with your hips. Keep your knees straight and your head back. Hold this position for five to 10 seconds, then push back to starting position. To feel more stretch, place your hands farther apart.

22. THIGH FIRMER AND KNEE STRETCH

Sit on the edge of your chair or lie on your back with your legs stretched out in front and your heels resting on the floor. Tighten the muscle that runs across the front of the knee by pulling your toes toward your head. Push the back of the knee down toward the floor so you also feel a stretch at the back of your knee and ankle. For a greater stretch, put your heel on a footstool and lean forward as you pull your toes toward your head.

out overstressing your joints and muscles are key elements in a successful program.

Endurance Exercises

Endurance or aerobic exercises are beneficial because they strengthen your heart and increase your lung efficiency. They also lessen fatigue by giving you more stamina so you can work longer without tiring as quickly. And endurance exercises help you sleep better, control your weight and lift your spirits.

Just about any exercise that uses the large muscles of the body in a continuous, rhythmic activity can be an endurance exercise, depending upon the person doing the exercise. For some, walking will increase fitness. Athletes, however, must exercise vigorously to achieve an improvement in aerobic fitness. The signs that you are exercising at conditioning level are:

• increased heart rate
• increased breathing
• feeling warmer and/or sweating.

Some of the most beneficial endurance exercises for people with fibromyalgia are walking, water exercise and using a stationary bicycle.

WALKING

Walking requires no special skills and is inexpensive. You can walk almost anytime and anywhere. And you can measure walking in blocks or time, so your progress is easy to monitor. However, you will need a good pair of supportive walking shoes. A great guide to help you develop a walking fitness routine is

Walk With Ease: Your Guide to Walking for Better Health, Improved Fitness and Less Pain ($8.95), available through the Arthritis Foundation Web site, www.arthritis.org, or by calling 800/207-8633. Arthritis Foundation books are also available at all bookstores.

The Talk Test

A simple way to tell if you're exercising at an appropriate level during aerobic activity, is known as the talk test. You should be able to carry on a conversation while exercising, without feeling out of breath. If you're unable to talk, slow down a bit, until you're working at a comfortable level.

Any exercise that uses your large muscles in a continuous, rhythmic activity can be an aerobic workout. Some examples include walking, bicycling, aerobic dance and water aerobics. The signs that you are exercising at an aerobic conditioning level are:

• Increased heart rate
• Increased breathing rate
• Increased body temperature or sweating

WATER EXERCISE

Swimming and exercising in warm water are especially good for stiff, sore muscles. Warm water between 84 and 88 degrees Fahrenheit helps relax your muscles and decrease pain. While you move your joints through their range of motion, water also helps support your body, putting less stress on your hips, knees and spine.

You can do warm-water exercises while standing in shoulder- or chest-high water or while sitting in shallow water. In deeper water, use an inflatable tube, flotation vest or belt to keep you afloat.

BICYCLING

Bicycling, especially on an indoor stationary bicycle, improves fitness without putting too much stress on your hips, knees and feet. Some stationary bicycles have the capacity to exercise your upper body as well. Adjust the seat height so that your knee straightens when the pedal is at the lowest point.

When you begin, do not pedal faster than 15 to 20 miles per hour or 60 revolutions per minute. Add resistance only after you have warmed up for five minutes. Don't add so much resistance that you have trouble pedaling. If cycling aggravates your pain, discuss this condition with your physician.

Increasing Your Fitness Level

The goal of aerobic activity should be to work within your target heart-rate range (see the chart, p. 85) for a total of 30 minutes at least three times a week whenever possible. It may take you a long time to work up to this ability level, so do not be discouraged. Within these parameters, you should be able to increase your fitness level steadily. The following section will give you some guidelines to help you determine whether you're working too hard or not hard enough.

UNDERSTANDING PERCEIVED EXERTION

When you are unsure of your pulse rate, try rating how hard you are working on a scale of zero to 10. Zero is equivalent to lying down and doing nothing. Ten is equal to working as hard as possible – very hard work that you could not do longer than seconds or minutes. Aim for moderate to strong exertion, somewhere between levels three and five.

FINDING YOUR TARGET HEART RATE

Find the target heart rate for your age group in the following chart, and use it as a guide. If your heart rate is higher than that suggested following peak exercise, slow down. When you work out at your suggested rate on a regular basis, your endurance and conditioning will improve.

However, if you are one of the 10 percent to 20 percent of fibromyalgia patients who have *mitral valve prolapse* – a condition that produces heart palpitations – or if you are just beginning to exercise, do not try to reach your target rate. Instead, speak to your doctor and exercise instructor about a pace that will be safe, yet still helpful. Keep your heart rate at the low end of the range. Consider the upper number a "not-to-exceed" heart rate.

You can measure your heart rate in beats per minute by counting your pulse for six seconds and adding a zero to that number (or by counting for 10 seconds and multiplying that number by six). For instance, if you count 20 beats in a 10-second period, your heart rate is six times 20, or 120 beats.

To find your wrist pulse, hold your arm with your palm up, facing you. Bend your hand slightly away from you. Place the tips of the index and middle fingers of your other hand on the center of your wrist, slightly

Finding Your Target Heart Rate

To find your target heart rate, you must stop during your activity and take your pulse. Keep walking or moving around to keep your blood circulating. Placing your index and middle fingers on your opposite wrist or below your jawline at your neck, count your pulse for six seconds and add a zero to that number (or count for 10 seconds and multiply by six). For example, if you count 14 beats in a 10-second period, your heart rate is six times 14, or 84 beats per minute.

Using the chart for a guide, find the target heart rate for your age group. You don't want your heart rate to be faster than the top end of the range during your aerobic exercise. If it does exceed the maximum, slow it down! If you are a beginner, consider the higher number in your range as a "not-to-exceed" heart rate. And take heart: if you exercise in your target range regularly, your endurance and conditioning will improve.

above the joint. Slide your fingertips toward the outside of your wrist (the thumb side), down over two tendons and into a soft depression between the tendons and the bone that run along the thumb side of your wrist. Apply gentle pressure in that depression, and you should feel the pulsation there, although it may take a little time to learn to feel it. It may be easier to find your pulse on one wrist than the other, so experiment.

Some people find it easier to feel their carotid pulse, located in the neck. To find this pulse, put the tips of your index and middle fingers behind your earlobe. Slide them straight down and below your jaw line. Apply gentle pressure; don't squeeze your neck between your thumb and fingers.

As you take your pulse, don't stop your workout entirely. It's important to keep your blood circulating. If possible, continue walking, cycling, or marching in place as you count. During water exercise, use a six-second heart rate, and your target heart rate will be the land heart rate minus 17.

Starting Your Exercise Program

Start your exercise program by asking your doctor for recommendations. He or she may recommend a regimen or may refer you to one of several different types of health professionals who can help you plan a realistic fitness program appropriate for your condition and abilities.

Physical therapists can show you special exercises to help keep your bones and muscles healthy and to increase your endurance.

Occupational therapists can explain how to do beneficial exercises for your hands, and they can show you how to perform daily activities properly so that you avoid fatigue and decrease stress on your body.

Other professionals who can assist you are physiatrists, health professionals who are members of the American College of Sports Medicine (ACSM), certified health and fitness instructors, personal trainers and exercise physiologists.

Contact your doctor, local hospital-sponsored fitness facility, health clinic or Arthritis Foundation chapter to learn about other exer-

Recommended Heart Rate Ranges

AGE	HEART RATE RANGE (60% - 75% of Age-Predicted Maximum Heart Rate)	10-SECOND COUNT
20	120 – 150	20 – 25
25	117 – 146	19 – 24
30	114 – 143	19 – 24
35	111 – 139	18 – 23
40	108 – 135	18 – 23
45	105 – 131	17 – 22
50	102 – 128	17 – 21
55	99 – 124	16 – 21
60	96 – 120	16 – 20
65	93 – 116	15 – 19
70	90 – 113	15 – 19
75	87 – 109	14 – 18
80	84 – 105	14 – 18
85	81 – 101	13 – 17
90	78 – 98	13 – 16

cise resources. Call 800/283-7800 or go to the Arthritis Foundation Web site at www.arthritis.org to find the local chapter near you.

STAYING MOTIVATED

If you find it difficult to keep yourself motivated, consider these approaches:

• Set a regular time or times during the day to exercise. Write it on your calendar to remind yourself. Refer to the "Goal Setting and Contracting" section in Chapter 7. Use the contract form there to set a realistic exercise goal. Write down what you plan to do and when you plan to do it. Have someone else sign the contract to help keep you motivated. Linking the time to something else helps make exercise a habit. For example, exercise daily before your morning shower,

before lunch or after reading the newspaper.
• Find a buddy to exercise with you. A companion can motivate you to exercise when you don't feel like it, and make exercising a more enjoyable, social experience.
• Stay in the habit of doing some exercise every day. On days when you aren't motivated, make an effort anyway. Interrupting the routine decreases your benefits and raises the chances that you'll abandon your program altogether.

MONITORING YOUR PROGRESS

Before you get too far into a fitness program, get a baseline fitness measurement by which you can set goals and evaluate your progress. You can measure your progress through the following techniques:
• See how far you can walk, bicycle or swim comfortably by measuring the distance on a marked running track, using the odometer on your car or bicycle to measure street distance, counting blocks or pool laps. Then measure how much more distance you cover over time.
• Measure how long it took you to cover a certain distance, for example, a number of blocks or pool lengths. Over time, try to cover the same course more quickly.
• Measure your heart rate, aiming to lower it over time.

Tips for Safe Exercise

Before exercise, do the following to maintain safe levels of fitness:
• Consult your physician or physical therapist before you begin a new fitness program.

• Warm up, and slowly increase the intensity of your exercise before starting any vigorous, endurance-type exercise. This warm-up period helps prevent injuries.
• Put on comfortable clothes. Your clothes should be loose and in layers so you can adapt to changes in temperature and activity. Breathable, easily washable fabrics are probably a good choice, too. There are many types of clothes made just for exercise, but you can wear your everyday, casual clothes if you prefer.
• Comfortable shoes are important for any exercise. Ill-fitting shoes can cause a number of problems in body mechanics. For instance, a good shoe will hold your foot in a normal position, which prevents your muscles, ligaments and tendons from straining to do that job. Your shoes should provide good support for the arches and position of your foot, and the soles should be made from non-slip, shock-absorbent material. Shock-absorbent insoles also can make exercise more comfortable.

During exercise, remember these tips:
• **Exercise at a comfortable, steady pace.** Don't work so hard that you are out of breath (see the Talk Test in this chapter). Give your muscles time to relax between each repetition. For increased range of motion and flexibility, do each exercise slowly and completely rather than attempting many rapid repetitions.
• **Breathe properly while you're working out.** People often hold their breath during exercise without realizing it. When possible, exhale upon muscle exertion, and inhale during muscle release. Counting out loud during

the exercise will help you breathe regularly. Don't try to breathe too deeply; just keep up your normal rate.

• **Don't do too much too quickly.** Building endurance should be a gradual process spread out over several weeks or months. You can gradually increase the number of repetitions of exercises you do as you get into shape.

• **Listen to your body.** You may need to tailor your exercise program on a daily basis, depending on how you feel. During the first few weeks, you may notice that your heart beats faster and you breathe faster when you exercise, and your muscles feel tense afterward. You may feel more tired at night, but you're likely to sleep better and more deeply than before. These are normal reactions to exercise that mean your body is adapting and getting into shape.

• **Stop exercising right away if you feel unpleasant symptoms.** These danger signs include chest tightness, severe shortness of breath, dizziness, faintness or nausea. If these symptoms occur, contact your doctor immediately. If you develop muscle pain or a cramp, gently rub and stretch the muscle. When the pain is gone, continue exercising with slow, easy movements. You may need to change your position or the way you are doing the exercise.

After exercise, it is important to:

• Cool down by doing your exercise activity at a slower, more relaxed pace for three to five minutes. For instance, if you've been walking briskly, slow down to a stroll. Also do gentle stretches to avoid stiff or sore muscles the next day. This practice helps your body cool, your heart slow down and your muscles relax.

• Don't stretch your muscles too much. Just stretch gently until you feel tension and then hold briefly.

• Massage any stiff or sore areas, or apply heat or cold treatments when necessary. Try soaking in a hot tub. Heat relaxes your joints and muscles and helps relieve pain. Cold also reduces pain and swelling for some people. Try placing a bag of frozen vegetables (such as peas or corn) over a sore area as a cold treatment.

MAKING EXERCISE A HABIT

We all can find many reasons not to exercise. Here are some of the most common reasons, along with ways to overcome them:

"I haven't exercised in so long. What if I can't do it?"

It's normal to feel hesitant about something you haven't done for a while. To overcome such feelings, try not to think of exercise as competition with others. Also, don't compare what you're able to do now with what you used to be able to do. Instead, focus on your current abilities. Do what you can. Each accomplishment, no matter how small, will help reinforce your confidence.

"I'm out of shape. It will take too long to see results."

Often, long-term problems can be addressed and managed by setting goals and writing out a contract. Refer to the Goal Setting and

Contracting information in Chapter 9, and follow those guidelines to make your own exercise contract.

"It hurts."

It's normal to have some soreness at first. Always warm up before exercise and cool down afterward to relax your muscles and reduce pain. Also, remember that exercise, in the long run, is likely to reduce the pain, fatigue and depression of fibromyalgia.

"My fibromyalgia is acting up."

Even when your fibromyalgia is active and your pain severe, don't skip your exercises entirely. Too much rest can be harmful, leading to stiffer and weaker muscles. Get plenty of rest, but also do range-of-motion exercises to help maintain your mobility. As your condition settles down, continue your range-of-motion exercises, and gradually return to your regular program.

"I don't have enough time."

Follow an exercise schedule. Several short exercise periods are just as good as one long period. Choose times that will not conflict with the work and family responsibilities that are important to you. Think of exercise as special time for yourself. Use it to think about other creative goals.

Once you begin to get into shape, you may actually find you have more time to exercise. With less pain, you can be more efficient.

"It's boring."

Do exercises you enjoy. Listen to music or an audio book while exercising. Exercise with friends or family members who understand your fibromyalgia. If you walk or bicycle, go to the park or another pleasant area.

"The weather's bad."

If you usually exercise with a group and can't get to your class in bad weather, do your exercises at home. (Keep some exercise equipment or exercise videotapes there.) If you swim or walk, have a back-up plan for indoors. For example, walk around a shopping mall, but don't stop to window shop.

"I don't like to exercise alone."

Ask friends or family members to exercise with you, or join an exercise class. Another option is to use one of the Arthritis Foundation's exercise videotapes to get the feeling of a group experience. Tapes are available for purchase from the Arthritis Foundation Web site, www.arthritis.org, or by calling 800/207-8633.

"It's too much work."

Maybe you're being too ambitious about your exercise program and trying to do too much. Relax. Enjoy the good feelings you have while you exercise and afterward. Exercising for fun is the best way to keep it up.

"My fibromyalgia isn't bothering me anymore."

Pain can be a good motivator. But don't slow down when the pain stops. Instead, vary your program with new and different exercises or activities.

Other exercise tips:
• Don't do vigorous exercises. If you notice more pain or are unable to do as much as you have been, talk to your doctor or physical therapist.
• If just one or two areas of your body are painful, adapt your exercises to put less stress on those areas. For example, if you are having more pain in your lower body (the weight-bearing area), switch from walking to water exercises, or try a resistance-free stationary bicycle.
• Keep track of your exercise routine by using an exercise diary. The following page is an example you can photocopy and use.

EXERCISE DIARY

Use this chart to keep records of your exercise activities.				
Date/Time	**Exercises**	**Frequency/ Duration**	**Perceived Exertion or Heart Rate**	**Feelings/ Comments**

Chapter 7

Eating Well:

Diet and Fibromyalgia

Can what you eat cause, cure or affect your fibromyalgia? Since symptoms of fibromyalgia can vary from day to day, it's natural to think that what you ate yesterday may have caused or reduced the pain you feel today.

Research has not yet proven that any specific foods affect fibromyalgia. But we do know that eating a good, balanced diet helps each body function at its best. Following a balanced diet can help you feel better, stay healthy, prevent chronic diseases such as some cancers and cardiovascular disease, and be a positive step toward managing your fibromyalgia.

Gradually Adopt a Good Diet

Eating well does not mean you have to starve yourself or eliminate the foods you love. It means making gradual changes that allow you to focus on healthful meals you enjoy. You are more likely to stick with these types of changes to achieve a healthier diet:

• reduce salt, fat, cholesterol, sugar and alcohol intake

• include fiber, fruits and vegetables, and calcium-rich foods.

A NOTE ON DIET "CURES"

You may read or hear about claims that special diets, supplements or foods cure health problems. Some of these claims are frauds. Others are unproven remedies (see Chapter 3). Consider diets unsafe and ineffective unless scientific tests prove them otherwise. Ask these questions:

• Does the diet eliminate any essential food group from the Food Guide Pyramid (discussed later in this chapter)?

• Does it stress only a few foods or eliminate certain foods?

• Does it claim to cure your fibromyalgia?

• Are its ads misleading, created to look like news articles instead of advertising?

• Do its claims lack scientific evidence such as published studies?

• Do you suspect that the diet could be harmful to your health?

If the answer is yes to any of these questions, avoid the diet. If you do suspect that certain foods are related to any of your symptoms, discuss your concerns with your doctor.

What Is a Good Diet?

Experts recommend five basic guidelines for a balanced, healthful diet. Use these in planning daily meals. The following sections explain how each of the guidelines is helpful.

EAT A VARIETY OF FOODS

Variety, balance and moderation are keys to a healthful diet. Variety usually means eating more grains, fruits and vegetables than most Americans do. A good diet includes some choices from each of five different groups of foods: breads and cereals, fruits, vegetables, dairy products and meats. Together they provide the 40 or more nutrients your body needs to grow and function.

Pain, fatigue and depression can lower your appetite or cause you to avoid foods that require time or effort to prepare. Follow the tips in the box below to make food preparation easier.

Health professionals in your community can help you learn more efficient cooking methods. For example, your doctor can refer you to an occupational therapist for advice on easier ways to cook. Some local chapters of the Arthritis Foundation and the cooperative Extension Services of some state

Making Meal Preparation Easier

Pain can reduce your appetite and make meal preparation more difficult. You may tend to avoid foods that take more time and effort to prepare. Here are a few ways that you can make meal preparation easier on your body so that it is easier to eat healthfully.

• Plan rest breaks during meal preparation.

• Use good posture to avoid pain during cooking tasks.

• Arrange your kitchen for convenience. Keep the tools you use most within easy reach.

• Buy healthy convenience foods, such as sliced and chopped vegetables.

• Add fresh fruit and bread to a frozen dinner for a simple, satisfying meal.

• Use kitchen appliances and tools that save you time and effort, such as electric can openers and microwave ovens.

• Share meals with friends or family members so you can split the cooking tasks and enjoy the company.

universities also may sponsor cooking classes or demonstrations. In addition, the Arthritis Foundation publishes a free brochure called "Diet and Your Arthritis," which provides some basic guidelines for achieving a healthy overall diet. Call 800/283-7800 or access the Arthritis Foundation Web site at www.arthritis.org to find your local chapter and receive other information.

Some medications can affect how well your body uses what you eat. For most people, eating a variety of foods will help keep up nutrient levels. Ask your physician how your medications affect your nutrition and whether a vitamin supplement may be useful.

EASE UP ON FAT AND CHOLESTEROL

Reducing fats and cholesterol in your diet may help prevent cardiovascular disease. The American Heart Association recommends that people limit fat intake to no more than 30 percent of their calories. Someone eating 2,000 calories a day, for instance, should eat only 67 fat grams a day or less. AHA recommends a cholesterol intake of less than 300 milligrams per day, the equivalent of about one and a half eggs.

Fat, a source of concentrated calories, contributes to extra pounds. To lower saturated fat and cholesterol, choose low-fat cuts of meat and low-fat dairy products. Reduce your servings of red meat and pork, and limit the use of added fats, oils, salad dressings, nuts and nut butters. A daily serving of red meat or pork the size of a deck of playing cards (approximately three ounces) is adequate for most adults.

EAT VEGETABLES, FRUITS AND WHOLE GRAINS

Carbohydrates are the basic energy supply for our bodies. Not all carbohydrates are equal, however. Simple carbohydrates, such as refined sugar and honey, contain few other nutrients. A candy bar will give you quick energy, but little else. We digest it quickly, which drives up our blood sugar and strains our insulin-producing pancreas. The boost of energy received by our bodies after eating candy bars doesn't last long.

Complex carbohydrates – fruits, vegetables and whole-grain products like high-fiber rolls – are digested more slowly, are low-fat and create a feeling of fullness, a help to any weight watcher. (Overeat either form of carbohydrate, however, and your body converts the excess to fat.) Eat a slice of whole wheat bread, for example, and you get energy but also vitamins, minerals, fiber and some protein. Fiber comes from parts of plants your body cannot digest. Some types of fibers result in softer stools, less constipation and more rapid elimination of waste. Fibers such as oat bran also help lower cholesterol levels. Fiber from foods is preferable to fiber from supplements, because you get the additional nutrients of foods like bran, fruits and vegetables.

SPARE THE SUGAR AND SALT

Too much sugar adds excess calories and promotes weight gain and tooth decay. When checking food labels for added sugar, look for the words dextrose, sucrose, fructose, honey and dextrin. Carbohydrates in general should make up 55 percent to 60 percent of your calories, and the bulk should come from complex carbohydrates such as vegetables, fruits and grains.

The American Heart Association suggests that you hold sodium intake to about 2,700 mg a day, or about 1 $^1/_4$ teaspoon of salt. Sodium causes your body to retain water and can affect your blood pressure. Many foods now come with low- or no-salt-added choices. This change makes it easier to maintain a low-sodium diet. Watch for excess sodium levels on prepared food labels.

DRINK ALCOHOL IN MODERATION

Excessive alcohol consumption can have many adverse effects on your health, including weakened bones, which can lead to osteoporosis. Alcohol adds unwanted pounds with extra, empty calories. It can also increase the *uric acid* in the body, increasing your susceptibility to a disease called *gout,* which is marked by pain and inflammation.

Alcohol does not mix well with certain medications used in treating fibromyalgia. For example, it can increase the sedative effect of tricyclic antidepressants and selective serotonin reuptake inhibitors (SSRIs), causing temporary mental impairment. Stomach problems also are more likely if you drink alcohol and take aspirin or other nonsteroidal anti-inflammatory drugs (NSAIDs). Large amounts of alcohol combined with acetaminophen can damage the liver. If you are taking any medications, check with your doctor or pharmacist about drinking alcohol, even in moderation.

THE FOOD GUIDE PYRAMID

The Food Guide Pyramid (see illustration), developed by the U.S. Department of Agriculture, shows how to follow healthy dietary guidelines and make wise food choices. Select most foods from the bottom two layers of the pyramid and fewer foods from the top, based on the recommended number of servings. The pyramid can guide you to a balanced diet with moderate amounts of sugar, sodium and saturated fat, and the right amount of calories to maintain a healthy weight.

THE FOOD LABELING ACT

With the Food Labeling Act of 1994, manufacturers of food products were required to provide a new, more comprehensive nutrition label on their packaging. Many products already listed ingredients, but there were no standards for comparing one food with another. The new labels allow you to evaluate the nutritional content of the food so you can make smart choices for a healthier diet.

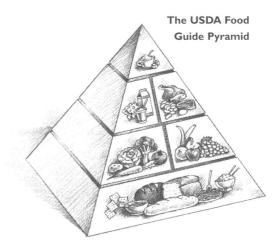

The USDA Food Guide Pyramid

The Food Labeling Act also set new guidelines for what health claims a food manufacturer can make. Claims such as "fat-free," "cholesterol-free," "low-sodium," and others now are defined by government standards. Certain requirements must be met for these claims to be made. Instead of learning what each claim means, remember these key words to help you judge nutritional content:

Light: A food has one-third fewer calories or half the fat of the standard version of the food (for example, light potato chips would have half the fat of standard potato chips). The sodium content of a low-calorie, low-fat food is reduced by 50 percent.

Low: You can eat a large amount of this food without exceeding the daily value for the particular nutrient that is described as "low."

Fat-free: The item contains less than 0.5 grams of fat per serving.

A fat-free food: The food naturally has no fat.

Lean: The fat content of meat is less than 10 grams of fat, less than 4 grams of saturated fat, and less than 95 milligrams of cholesterol per serving and per 100 grams.

Extra-lean: The fat content of meat is less than 5 grams of fat, less than 2 grams of saturated fat, and less than 95 milligrams of cholesterol per serving and per 100 grams.

High: One serving of the food contains 20 percent or more of the daily value for the nutrient being described (such as calcium).

Good source: One serving of the food contains 10 percent to 19 percent of the daily value for the nutrient being described.

NUTRITION RESOURCES

Many information resources can answer your questions about your diet. One place to start is with your doctor. He or she can refer you to experts in diet and nutrition for help with applying diet guidelines, planning a weight-loss program or answering any of your questions.

Here are some other tips:

• Check with local hospitals, health clinics and public health departments, which often have individual nutritional counseling and weight-reduction groups.

• Search for a registered dietitian or a nutritionist in the Yellow Pages of the telephone directory or by asking your doctor.

• Call the Consumer Information Center at 800/688-9889 to request a copy of "USDA's Food Guide Pyramid," a colorful, easy-to-read, 30-page booklet. (Cost is $1.) Or, search the CIC's Web site at www.pueblo.gsa.gov.

• Contact the Cooperative Extension Service for answers to your questions about meal planning. Look under the "Government Offices" section of your phone book.

• Contact other voluntary health and professional organizations that promote a healthy diet, such as local chapters of the American Heart Association, American Cancer Society, American Diabetes Association and American Dietetic Association.

• Check your bookstore or library for relevant, recently published books on diet, weight loss or general nutrition.

Chapter 8

Getting Along:

Developing and Maintaining Relationships

Some studies show that people with chronic conditions who don't have a strong support network are likely to have more pain, be less active, use more medication and feel more depressed, helpless and anxious than those with a support network. Close relationships with others can have a positive effect on your psychological and physical well-being.

How well a family copes when faced with health problems depends on their pre-fibromyalgia relationships. Some families pull closer together, united in their determination, and maintain an environment supportive of every member. But some families sag under the weight of a chronic illness and splinter apart.

Your Relationships With Others

In Gregg Piburn's 1999 book *Beyond Chaos: One Man's Journey Alongside His Chronically Ill Wife* (Arthritis Foundation), the author describes the challenges of coping with his wife Sherrie's fibromyalgia, and the impact her illness has had on his emotional well-being and their relationship:

I left a cozy corporate job in 1991 to start a one-person consulting business. "You are crazy," said a former co-worker who dedicates his life to comfort, planning and predictability. I could easily live with such a bland person calling me crazy. However, I read into his numerous comments that I was crazy AND selfish. I told him I had longed for years to be my own boss. I finally had a chance to make this lifelong dream a reality but, as my friend pointed out, the seed of that dream came to life before chronic illness put a whammy on Sherrie. I not only had to wrestle with whether I could achieve business success on my own, I also had to overcome strong feelings of guilt.

Author Anthony de Mello said: "In life, one plays the hand one is dealt to the best of one's ability. Those who insist on playing not the hand they were given, but the one they insist they should have been dealt, these are life's failures. We are not asked if we will play; that is not an option. Play we must; the option is how."

Sherrie did not maliciously choose to become chronically ill. I did not decide to remain physically healthy to spite her. Fate dealt Sherrie and I the hand that led to our current situation. For numerous reasons, this hand called chronic illness comes loaded with wild cards called guilt. Neither of us need feel guilty.

Feelings of resentment, guilt and frustration are common in families of people with fibromyalgia. There are ways to cope with these feelings and to maintain healthy relationships. Here are a few key elements to successfully managing a chronic illness in your family:

• **Communication.** By sharing thoughts and feelings, family members gain a better understanding of each other's expectations and needs.

• **Tolerance.** By maintaining respect for each other's limitations, family members are less likely to have emotional blowouts.

• **Humor.** A sense of humor can make any burden a little lighter.

• **Support.** Successful families are available to provide help and support regardless of the circumstances.

Communication skills can be a vital tool in your relationships with your family and close friends, particularly now that fibromyalgia is part of the picture. This chapter will help you deal with loved ones, friends, business associates or health-care professionals.

Communication: Using "I" Messages

When people are annoyed or frustrated, they often express their feelings too aggressively, putting other people on the defensive. Or they reveal their feelings too passively, clamming up and holding a grudge. It's easy to slip into using what psychologists call "you" messages: "Why do *you* always make us late?" "*You* don't understand how I feel." "*You* really make me angry when you do that."

"You" messages can seem like an attack to recipients. Their natural reaction is to become defensive. Now both you and the other person are bearing your verbal fists, and the situation may escalate into an argument and bad feelings. Your message is lost in the transaction.

A better way to communicate is to use "I" messages. These are factual statements of how you feel; they don't accuse or blame the other person. When you say, "I get upset when I'm late," or "I am angry that you did that," the other person can respond to the content of what you've said, rather than defending against an attack.

Consider the following examples of a discussion using "you" messages:

Person 1: "I wish you would help. You're going to make us late. Help or stay out of my way."

Person 2: "Hey, why are you always criticizing me? You find fault with everything I do."

Person 1: "I'm criticizing you? You're criticizing me – and that's what you always do."

Now, consider the same discussion that contains "I" statements:

Personally Speaking   Stories from real people with fibromyalgia

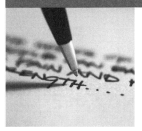

"At 30, I had surgery for a ruptured disc in my lower back. From that point on, I had bouts of pain that came and went pretty much like the weather. Ten years and several surgeries later, a neurologist diagnosed me with fibromyalgia. Since then, I've had major back surgery and developed a painful spinal condition called arachnoiditis. Now I can't tell which symptoms come from what condition.

The Bumpy Road to a Better Self
Ann B. McPherson
Kill Devil Hills, NC

"These days, I'm not able to walk or stretch. Stretching my spine causes more pain, and I've been having so many problems with my legs that I've stopped my regular walks. I'm on total rest. It can feel discouraging, but my husband is a rock. I said to him, 'I have not done one thing today, and I can hardly get around.' He said, 'Well, you went through a lot of stress last week, and that's set you back.' How many husbands would take the time to put all that together?

"Without the support of my family, I wouldn't have gotten this far. My daughter sent me a card that says, 'Mom, watching you as I have grown up, I know you have a real strength in your faith and in your belief in yourself, and that's gotten you as far as you have.' I looked at that card and said, 'This one's a keeper.'

"My spirits aren't always up. But I believe the Lord has a purpose for everything. The road I've gone down has really been a bumpy one, and it's not the one I would have chosen. But now that I've gone down it, I'm grateful for the person this experience has made me. I'm a much better person. I'm more compassionate, more giving. And I appreciate the sunshine."

Person 1: "Being late makes me uncomfortable. It's difficult enough for me to get ready because of my fibromyalgia. There must be some way we can speed things up."

Person 2: "It's difficult for me too, because I never know when offering help is the right thing to do."

Person 1: "Oh, I never thought of that. I'll tell you what: When I need your help in the future, I'll ask."

Person 2: "Great. That will make me feel better too."

- **Listen to yourself and others.** "I" messages take practice. Start by listening and practice changing each "you" message you hear to an "I" message in your head. The exercise soon will translate to your own expressions.

- **Keep trying.** If "you" messages and assigning blame have been your typical way of communicating, the other person may not hear the "I" messages right away. Keep using them anyway, and eventually the other person will hear you.

• **Don't manipulate.** "I" messages should report honest feelings. When used to manipulate the other person, communication will get worse.

• **Express positive feelings, too.** "I" messages are wonderful for expressing positive feelings and compliments.

LEARNING TO LISTEN

Listening is a crucial element of good communication. But many people are not good listeners because they don't know how to practice *active* listening. They assume listening is passive – they may hear the words but fail to understand the meaning. To become a good listener, practice the skill of active listening.

Here's what's involved:

• **Look interested.** Use nonverbal clues to show you're listening. Make eye contact, keep your posture relaxed, lean forward, use appropriate facial expressions (smile or look sympathetic), nod your head to show you are listening, and touch the person (if appropriate).

• **Sound like you are interested.** Encourage the speaker to continue with brief phrases or words: "Mm-hmm," "Oh?," "Go on," "Then what?" "Would you like to talk about it?"

• **Acknowledge the content of what you just heard.** Instead of responding with advice or information, first show that you understood the meaning of the other person's message by rephrasing what you think the speaker meant.

If what you say is not what he was trying to communicate, you've provided an opportunity for correction.

• **Acknowledge the speaker's emotional state.** People communicate their feelings by tone of voice, facial expression and other nonverbal cues. Simply saying "you sound sad/glad/ angry/scared" communicates your understanding, concern and acceptance of the person's feelings. Often these words encourage an even more open exchange.

GET THE DATA YOU NEED

A computer cannot process data it doesn't have – and neither can you. If you don't have enough information, you can't respond appropriately. How do you get a person to communicate more deeply and clearly?

• **Ask for more information.** Be honest if you are confused or think you missed the point: "I don't understand." "Would you say that another way?" "What do you mean?" "Please expand on that." "Tell me more."

• **Ask about meaning.** Sometimes there's a gap between what a person says and what he or she means. Paraphrasing is a good way to be sure you understood what the person meant. Be careful to paraphrase as a question, though. People don't like to be told what they meant. "You're telling me..." sounds like an accusation, and the response is likely to be anger or frustration because you didn't understand. "Are you saying...?" promotes further clarification.

• **Be specific.** We often speak in generalities when specifics would be more helpful. A question like "How do you feel?" may not elicit a useful answer if you want to know something specific. Better choices might be "Are you upset?" or "Does your head still hurt?" or "Is the room warm enough?"

COMMUNITY RESOURCES AND SELF-HELP GROUPS

Relationships with friends and family aren't the only ones you can build on. Many communities, for example, have Arthritis Foundation chapters that offer the Fibromyalgia Self-Help Course, a course designed to show people with fibromyalgia how to self-manage their condition. This course will not only educate you further about fibromyalgia, but also will help you form a supportive network of individuals who share the condition. To find your local Arthritis Foundation chapter, call 800/283-7800, or log on to www.arthritis.org.

Of course, you can join any number of groups, including exercise groups, volunteer activities, art classes and book clubs that have nothing to do with fibromyalgia, but that may help you form the support network you need.

Sexuality and Fibromyalgia

Fibromyalgia can affect one's sexuality in a number of ways, especially because sexuality is not limited to physical activity. Sexuality includes one's feelings of attractiveness, desire for emotional closeness and openness to sensory experiences.

In fact, it's not unusual for a couple to experience communication and/or relationship difficulties when one partner has fibromyalgia. Part of the problem may stem from the depression and slump in self-esteem that can accompany changes in physical capabilities. And of course, it's hard to feel sexy when you are in pain or constantly fatigued.

A withdrawal from sex, coupled with a reluctance to discuss sexual needs and/or problems, can jeopardize your relationship. Your partner may misinterpret withdrawal as rejection, leading to a deterioration of your relationship.

To improve your sexual relationship, talk with your partner about your needs, desires and ideas. Learn to use communication skills (see "Communication: Using 'I' Messages" on page 98) to ask for what you need, to set boundaries and to let your partner know what feels good to you. Encourage your partner to express intimate feelings as well. He or she may be concerned that sexual activity is painful for you and thus feel anxious about intimacy. Avoiding sex, however, could create tension between you.

HOW FIBROMYALGIA AFFECTS YOUR SEX LIFE

Fibromyalgia can cause a variety of physical problems that may affect sexuality. Here are some of the more common problems and some tips to minimize them:

Fatigue:
• Plan sexual activity for when you are rested and relaxed.
• Plan ahead by pacing daily activities to avoid extreme fatigue in the evening.

How To Talk With Your Partner About Sex

Fibromyalgia may affect your sexual desire and your approach to sexual activity. Talking with your partner can help make you feel better and improve your relationship. Think about the following questions and discuss them with your partner:

- Has fibromyalgia altered your sexual relationship or your feelings about sex?
- What, if anything, has changed?
- What is more or less the same?
- Are there any sexual activities that are not as pleasant as they used to be?
- Are there any that are more enjoyable?
- Does lovemaking cause any particular problems for you or your partner?
- Where on your body do you enjoy being touched? Where is touching unpleasant?
- Are there new things you would like to try? If so, what are they?
- Have you talked to your partner about any of these things?

Adapted from *Celebrate Life: New Attitudes for Living with Chronic Illness*, The Arthritis Foundation, 1999

Pain and Muscle Stiffness:

- Try stretching activities to reduce stiffness.
- Take a warm bath or shower before sex to reduce pain.
- Find a more comfortable position. Communicate with your partner about what positions might be more comfortable for you. Speak up if the position you have been using is causing you pain or discomfort.

Medications:

- Some medications can have side effects that may decrease sexual drive. For example, some SSRIs, such as *Prozac,* can suppress orgasms and desire for sex. Consult your doctor if you are concerned about your medication's side effects.

Sexual fulfillment can be achieved in many ways, and it is up to you and your partner to find the right way for you. A person with fibromyalgia may find it necessary to adapt sexual activity but can still experience a close, intimate relationship. To learn new approaches to sex when you have a chronic illness, contact the Arthritis Foundation for a copy of the organization's free brochure, *The Arthritis Foundation's Guide to Intimacy.* Call 800/207-8633 for information.

Uplifting Activities

Doing uplifting activities can help balance the hassles and problems that lead to stress, depression, pain and fatigue. Choose to take time to have fun and enjoy yourself.

We aren't always taught how to nourish ourselves emotionally or spiritually. Sometimes, people are taught to do exactly the opposite: to silence their emotions and feelings. Nourishment of the mind and spirit can take many forms, such as laughing, crying, singing, listening to music, meditation, praying, enjoying nature, exercising or reading. Use the Uplifts Scale on p. 153 to help you track events that make you feel good. Try some of the group activities listed on the following pages.

WORKSHEET: Problem Solving

1. Select a current problem or concern and list any known causes.
2. Write down several possible solutions for dealing with this problem or its causes.
3. Consider the advantages and disadvantages of each option.
4. Select an option to try.
5. Evaluate your results after implementing the option selected.

1. PROBLEM/CAUSE

2. POSSIBLE SOLUTIONS	3. ADVANTAGES	DISADVANTAGES

4. OPTION TO TRY   5. RESULTS/OUTCOME

Part Four

Assume Responsibility
for What You Can Control

Chapter 9

In Control:

Your Role as a Self-Manager

When you're ill, it's sometimes easy to become passive, allowing others to make decisions and do things for you. When you have fibromyalgia, that attitude could be a critical mistake. Therapy begins with action, first by learning about your condition, and then by doing something about it. Promote yourself to executive manager of your condition.

This chapter can help you sort out your priorities, such as how to control your physical symptoms as much as possible, meet the emotional challenges of fibromyalgia and live a full life.

Five Habits of Successful Self-Managers

People who lead healthy lives with fibromyalgia have found innumerable, ingenious methods of dealing with the syndrome, some of which you'll read about in this book. Following are five tasks to help you become a successful self-manager of your fibromyalgia.

1. Learn All You Can About Fibromyalgia

Keep informed about fibromyalgia by asking your health-care professionals questions and reading as much about fibromyalgia as you can. This book is just one resource. Visit your local library and bookstore for others.

Check with local hospitals, health-maintenance organizations (HMOs), or other health-care facilities to find out what resources, such as classes and support groups, are available in your community.

Find your local chapter of the Arthritis Foundation by calling 800/283-7800 or checking the Web site at www.arthritis.org. The Arthritis Foundation's many local chapters and branches will have information on resources in your area, such as water-exercise classes and support groups for people with fibromyalgia. The Resources section at the end of this book contains more information about the Arthritis Foundation's many services.

2. Join Your Health-Care Team

If you don't have a doctor, get one immediately. (See "Finding a Physician" in Chapter 4.)

Then become an active, not passive, member of the team that is treating your fibromyalgia.

Take part in planning your treatment program and follow it. Remember that fibromyalgia treatment includes not only medication, but also exercise, stretching and adequate rest.

Write down questions, symptoms, problems and concerns to ask your doctor so you don't forget them when you're at your appointment. Be brief and concise.

Monitor your symptoms and report any changes to your doctor. For a full explanation of how to interact with your health-care team, see Chapter 4.

3. Develop a Healthy Lifestyle

If you don't feel healthy, imitate the habits of a healthy person. You may find that the feeling rubs off.

• Exercise regularly.

• Eat a balanced diet of tasty, healthy foods. See Chapter 7 for more information on a healthy diet.

• Get plenty of rest.

• Do things that make you happy and your life richer.

• Adopt a positive attitude.

4. Assume Responsibility for What You Can Control

Having a healthy mind and body begins by taking responsibility for yourself. You are the only person who has control over your thoughts and actions. Good living with fibromyalgia requires committing yourself to doing everything you can to get better. Don't just take the medications your doctor prescribes. Find more ways to relieve your symptoms. Try exercising, eating

a healthy diet and meditating to relax. Three basic skills can help you maintain independence:

• Set goals and work toward them (see "Goal Setting and Contracting" later in this chapter).

• Get help when you need it. Try brainstorming with family and friends, or use the problem-solving techniques in this chapter. Ask questions, read a book or seek professional guidance when you've exhausted your own methods of overcoming an obstacle.

• Accept what you can't control. Some problems and symptoms are not going to go away. You will have to find a way to come to terms with them.

5. Master Emotional Challenges

Practice stress-reduction and relaxation exercises. Besides promoting a pleasant, comfortable state of well-being, relaxation helps your body to rest and rebuild. See Chapter 13 for stress-reduction tips.

Discuss your feelings and problems with family and friends so they know what you're experiencing and so they can offer assistance and understanding.

Educate your family and friends about fibromyalgia. Share articles or books. If they have questions, meet together with your physician or another member of your health-care team.

Seek outside counseling or help if your problems seem overwhelming. Many sources of counseling exist in every community. In addition, there are non-profit organizations that may offer assistance to people with chronic illnesses, such as rides to the doctor. Keep searching until you find the help that fits your needs.

Personally Speaking Stories from real people with fibromyalgia

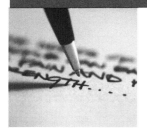

"Itravel through life like everyone else, but I happen to have fibromyalgia. Don't call me a fibromyalgic, because that word gives this syndrome total control over me, the person. My quest is to cross the fibromyalgia maze to find ways to feel that I am in control, not my fibromyalgia. Of the many people I've talked to who also have fibromyalgia, the ones in despair are the people who have lost their perception of control over their lives.

To Be or Not To Be... In Control
Ann Jensen
Powell, OH

"How do I seize control? First, I develop personal goals and pleasures. What gives you pleasure? If you're like me, you have almost forgotten. But start small: sitting in a sunny spot at home, reading a mystery, watching the sunset, praying, calling an upbeat friend or taking a warm bath. When you have listed your small pleasures, continue toward the grander ones, such as lunch with friends, concerts, traveling. List the things that put pleasure back in your life.

"To achieve this list of pleasure goals, start tiny once again. Turn the dial off on the 'it's all in your head' and 'it's only stress' friends. Educate yourself on fibromyalgia rather than depending on your doctor alone. List the things you are thankful for. Practice deep breathing, try a cat stretch or listen to a relaxation tape. Listening to these tapes taught me how tightly I held myself. Perhaps the plan seems simple, but it proves you are in control and heading down the right road.

"Don't stop. Write down a stretching routine, not just to stretch, but exhaling to relax until you feel that foreign sense of 'relaxed' muscles. Don't count; just gently hold the stretch until you've achieved some release.

"Add walking, water aerobics and strengthening. Add them very gently, and remember that 'no pain, no gain' is not true – it's barbaric torture. Try five minutes a day, then 10, 15 and 20; three times a week, then four, then five. How fast and furiously you exercise is your decision. I have a need to be accountable to a piece of paper, so I check off my successes (or setbacks) every day.

"I encourage you to create a list of personal goals and a feasible plan of attack to put you in control, and then accomplish each step. Setbacks and flares happen. Just pull up at your mental bed-and-breakfast, and ride them out; then cruise on to your own perception of control and hope. The alternative is to do nothing and flirt with despair."

Contract Form

THIS WEEK I WILL: _____ **WEEK OF:** _____

For Example: This week I will <u>walk</u> <u>around the block</u> <u>before lunch</u> <u>three times</u>.

                      (WHAT)   (HOW MUCH)   (WHEN)   (HOW MANY)

What

How Much

When

How Many Days

How Certain Are You *(On a scale of 0 to 10 with 0 being totally unsure and 10 being totally confident)*

Signature:

Goal-Setting and Contracting

Like the manager of a business or organization, you must first know what you want to accomplish before charting a course of action. Goal setting can help you decide what's important in managing fibromyalgia.

Think of a goal as something you would like to accomplish in the next three to six months. Be realistic and specific. Start by thinking of all the things you would like to do. Then, decide which of those things can be done in the next several weeks or months. If you choose a goal that is too difficult to achieve, you may get discouraged and give up.

Goals usually need to be broken down into small, manageable steps or tasks. For example, if your overall goal is to improve your physical fitness, try these steps:

• Make an appointment to see your doctor or physical therapist to get information on the types of exercise that would be best for your condition.

• Research classes such as warm-water swimming classes or adaptive physical-education classes at the local Arthritis Foundation chapter, hospital, community college or health club.

- Find a friend to exercise with.
- The next step is to get started. Decide which steps to work on and create a plan for accomplishing these goals.

Activity: Contracting for a Better Life With Fibromyalgia

To map out a schedule for accomplishing your goals, draw up a weekly contract with yourself. Key parts of such a contract include specific steps toward your overall goal and specific plans about how you will fulfill your plan. For example: What will you do? List a specific behavior or activity such as walking. How often will you walk? List the times per week you intend to walk. How long will you walk? List the duration of your walk. When will you walk? List the time of day you will walk or at what point in the day (such as before lunch) you will walk.

An example of your goal: "Three times this week I will walk for 10 minutes before lunch."

Start slowly. Limit your contracts to something you can do in one week. And don't begin with a contract to do things every day; three to four times a week is more realistic.

Assess your confidence in your project using a scale of zero to 10 (on which zero is unsure and 10 is confident), and rate your certainty about completing the contract. You should have a confidence level of seven or more.

Make copies of the Contract Form on the previous page to keep a record of your weekly goals.

To stay motivated, have someone else – a family member, a friend, or perhaps a member of your health-care team – sign the contract.

PROBLEM SOLVING

Problem-solving skills are essential to meeting your goals and setting realistic contracts. Try the Problem-Solving Worksheet on page 112 if you're having trouble overcoming obstacles.

Activity: Creating a Problem-Solving Worksheet

1. Identify a problem fibromyalgia has caused in your life. What are your concerns? What's causing them? Can the problem be broken down into smaller, more manageable issues? For example:
"Early mornings are bad."
– Why?
"Because I never feel well until I'm at the office for a couple of hours."
– When is it worst?
"When I'm responsible for the car pool because I have to get up even earlier."
2. List ideas to solve the problem. What do you want to achieve, and how can you do that? Write down as many options as you can. Ask for suggestions from family, friends, members of your health-care team or community resources. For example: "I could take a hot bath for stiffness. Or dress more warmly."

Problem-Solving Worksheet

- Select a current problem or concern, and list any known causes.

- Write down several possible solutions.

- Consider the advantages and disadvantages of each option.

- Select an option to try.

- Evaluate your results.

"I could check with my doctor on new medications."

"I could drop out of the Thursday night book club."

"I could check with my supervisor to see if I could work out a 'flex-time' schedule, beginning and ending my day later."

3. Consider the pros and cons. What are the consequences of each option? What are the advantages and disadvantages? Rank their order from least to most practical and desirable. Example:

"Taking a hot bath would mean getting up even earlier."

"Dressing more warmly doesn't always help."

"The doctor recently gave me a new medication, and I want to give it a fair trial before switching it."

"Dropping out of the Thursday night book club means I won't enjoy this discussion, but then I can stay home and relax on Thursday nights. Perhaps I can go once a month instead."

"My supervisor might be open to having me come in later and stay later. She's often had trouble finding people to finish up last-minute items."

4. Select one option and develop a plan to implement it. Example:

"I'll ask my supervisor about it. She's usually most receptive to new ideas right around the mid-morning coffee break."

5. Put your plan into action. Remember that change can be difficult and give your idea a chance before deciding it won't work.

6. Evaluate the results. Has your problem been solved? Are you headed in the right direction? If not, choose another idea from your list and try again. Example:

"After I switched to flex-time, there were trade-offs I hadn't foreseen. It's too late to go out after work, and I have to miss the evening news. Sometimes I'm so tired when I get home, I'm out with the lights.

"But overall, it's been worth it. My body has a couple of hours to loosen up before work, and I almost feel like a human being when I get there."

7. Accept that the problem may not be solved immediately. If your ideas don't work now, try them again later. Don't feel discouraged. Keep going, and look for alternate paths to what you want to accomplish.

Recording Your Experiences

Why is keeping a journal so helpful? In *Opening Up: The Healing Power of Confiding in Others*, author James W. Pennebaker, PhD, a professor of psychology at the University of Texas at Austin, showed that people with chronic illness who wrote about their painful feelings and losses reported fewer symptoms, fewer visits to the doctor, fewer days off

Personally Speaking Stories from real people with fibromyalgia

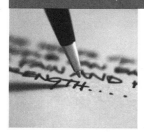

"It has been my experience that living with fibromyalgia is teaching me a great lesson in discipline. Of course I don't mean to say that my former lack of discipline is in any way responsible for my having fibromyalgia. It just so happens that having fibromyalgia has given me something positive in my life. My improved discipline is wonderful. To think that what mostly seems like an unfair situation can bring about something positive in our lives.

A Lesson in Discipline
Kerry Freyne Kennedy
Atlanta, GA

"When I first began to suffer with fibromyalgia, my chief defect — my lack of discipline — was still alive and well. Slowly I began to learn that without discipline the quality of my life with fibromyalgia would not improve. Suddenly I found myself saying, 'Well I just have to... keep writing that journal in order to assess what makes me feel better and what aggravates the fibromyalgia... just get up and do those stretches no matter how much pain I'm in, because invariably it makes me feel better... keep talking to others who have fibromyalgia because it helps me, and I help them... keep going with that healthy diet because it makes me feel better... keep understanding that a flare is just a silly old flare, and it's not going to last forever...'

"To do what's necessary to feel better takes discipline, and for those of us who have fibromyalgia, I promise that such discipline is well-rewarded in many ways. It puts you in charge of your life and your condition, and every positive thing you can do on a daily basis to help yourself gives you a feeling of strength and pride at the end of the day. I know it's difficult and at times seems almost impossible, but as we draw from our own inner strength and our faith we find that each day we have more and more discipline to go on and make the best of it in a positive way. So here's to us and our strength. Let's always keep our faces to the sun."

work, improved mood and outlook, and even enhanced immune system function.

Keeping records of your experiences with fibromyalgia can make a difference in your health. Many people find it useful to write about those experiences in a journal or diary, along with other observations. You may also find it helpful to share them with your physi-

cian or health-care professional. A written record of your experiences, whether a journal, diary or self-monitoring worksheet, can:
• provide you and your doctor with concrete documentation of your symptoms
• help you to communicate with doctors, family members, friends, co-workers or employers

• help you understand your disease more fully and identify your symptom patterns
• identify factors that trigger symptoms and fluctuations
• serve as a more objective memory aid
• help you integrate your feelings about your symptoms and focus on healing
• help you reassert control

Activity: Keeping a Journal

On the following pages, you will find different methods for recording your symptoms and experiences with fibromyalgia. These methods include a Symptoms Diary, a Sample Thoughts Diary and a weekly Time Analysis Worksheet. Try different techniques until you find one that's practical and easy to use.

Here are some guidelines for writing and recording your symptoms and experiences. Monitor only what is important to you, not what you think you ought to care about. Below are some factors to consider:
• amount/location of pain
• level of energy/fatigue
• hours of sleep/rest
• medications and their side effects
• unusual symptoms
• stress/problems
• exercise
• activity level
• food intake
• weight
• positive experiences
• mood changes
• thoughts/reactions to daily events
• something funny you saw or heard that day

Keeping a journal, like any new habit, will take a while to feel natural. To give it a fair trial, set a schedule for writing in your journal. For example, set aside five to 10 minutes, three times a week. If you like it, you'll probably find yourself writing on a regular basis. Select a method that fits your schedule and needs. Here are a few strategies:
• Record a symptom log in a calendar, diary or notebook. Enter symptoms daily or weekly as needed during flares or times of uncertainty.
• Write (or use a typewriter, computer or tape recorder if handwriting is too painful) about your experiences with fibromyalgia and your reactions to these experiences. One woman simply started writing down all her disease symptoms along with her deepest feelings and thoughts about her condition.
• Divide a sheet of paper in half, and on one side record all of the facts of the day: problems, challenges or positive experiences. On the other side, record your emotional reactions and thoughts about these events. Logs like these are useful for emotional release and self-discovery.
• Select only a few symptoms to monitor initially, such as pain, fatigue and mood. Use a Symptoms Diary to keep track of changes. A tool that shows how symptoms change can help you see the relationships between symptoms.
• Date your entries so that you can look back over them and see patterns and progress.
• Write freely and selfishly. Don't worry about grammar or misspellings. Keep this diary to yourself; you'll write more honestly.

Write to develop insight into your feelings and to provide an emotional release.

Use a journal printed for recording these feelings and experiences. The Arthritis Foundation publishes a journal for this purpose called *Toward Healthy Living: A Wellness Journal*. This spiral-bound, beautifully illustrated book contains daily trackers for pain and mood. To order, call 800-207-8633 or log on to the Foundation Web site at www.arthritis.org.

Thoughts Diary

To appreciate the power of your self-talk and the part it plays in your emotional life, make your own thoughts diary. Make a notation each time you experience an unpleasant emotion. Include everything you tell yourself to keep the emotion going.

DATE	UNPLEASANT EMOTION	SITUATION	SELF-TALK	RATIONAL RESPONSE

Symptoms Diary

It is useful to monitor your pain level and mood to learn more about possible associations. Use the chart below to rate your current mood and pain level on the 0-10 scale. For the next week, rate your pain and mood three times per day (e.g. AM — when you get up in the morning, Midday and PM — before going to bed). Then look for patterns or possible associations.

FOR EACH TIME PERIOD
- Mark an **X** across from the number that describes your **mood**; (0=best mood, 10=worst mood or most anxious/depressed/negative feelings).
- Mark an **0** across from the rating of **pain**; (0=no pain, 10=worst pain).

MOOD/PAIN DIARY

	AM	Mid-Day	PM	AM	Mid-Day	PM	AM	Mid-Day	PM	AM	Mid-Day	PM	AM	Mid-Day	PM	AM	Mid-Day	PM	AM	Mid-Day	PM
10																					
9																					
8																					
7																					
6																					
5																					
4																					
3																					
2																					
1																					
0																					
	Mon/Day 1			Tue/Day 2			Wed/Day 3			Thur/Day 4			Fri/Day 5			Sat/Day 6			Sun/Day 7		

Symptoms Diary

Use the following worksheet to help you analyze how you spend a typical week.

	MON	TUE	WED	THUR	FRI	SAT	SUN
6 a.m.							
7 a.m.							
8 a.m.							
9 a.m.							
10 a.m.							
11 a.m.							
noon							
1 p.m.							
2 p.m.							
3 p.m.							
4 p.m.							
5 p.m.							
6 p.m.							
7 p.m.							
8 p.m.							
9 p.m.							
10 p.m.							
11 p.m.							
midnight							

Chapter 10

Closing the Gates:

Ways To Manage Pain

People with fibromyalgia feel chronic, or persistent, pain in their muscles all over their bodies. Even a stimulus that other people would hardly notice – such as someone pressing your skin with their finger – feels painful. They may have headaches or stomach distress, tingling feelings, sensitivity to hot and cold, and painful stomach cramps. The variety and range of pain they may feel is disheartening and exhausting. Outside factors may worsen pain for someone with fibromyalgia. One stressful situation can trigger a downward spiral of diminishing health.

Thankfully, there are ways to manage pain. Although the methods discussed in this chapter can't make the pain disappear completely, they may be valuable in helping people with fibromyalgia manage their pain more effectively.

Methods for Managing Pain

For most people with fibromyalgia, medication for pain is limited to aspirin, other over-the-counter NSAIDs or the analgesic acetaminophen, providing only minor relief. Antidepressants that promote the release of serotonin may ease pain and facilitate sleep, thus breaking the pain-fatigue cycle. (However, SSRIs like *Prozac* may disturb sleep, especially if taken at bedtime.) Narcotic painkillers (used in conjunction with a comprehensive treatment program that includes exercise, education, medications for sleep and depression, and counseling) may help those people for whom nothing else works. For a full explanation of medications, see Chapter 2.

Other measures besides your doctor's prescriptions may help you manage your pain, however. The following chapters describe some of these measures. In addition to this chapter on pain, the rest of the book gives guidance on how to deal with fatigue, get a better night's sleep and manage stress.

What Is Pain?

Pain is your body's alarm system, signaling your brain that something is wrong. When part of your body is injured or damaged, nerves in that area release chemical signals. The nerves act like tiny telephone wires and

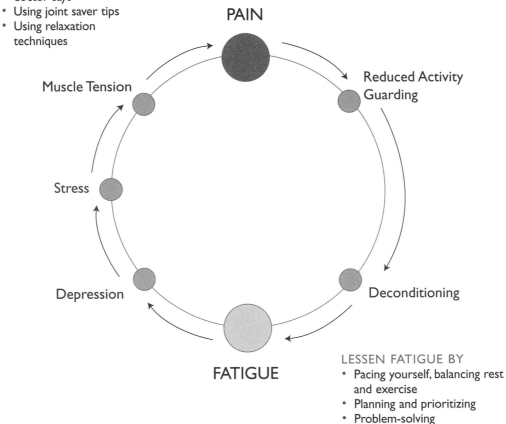

LESSEN PAIN BY
- Exercising
- Putting heat or cold on sore joints
- Taking your medications as your doctor says
- Using joint saver tips
- Using relaxation techniques

PAIN

Reduced Activity Guarding

Muscle Tension

Deconditioning

Stress

Depression

FATIGUE

LESSEN FATIGUE BY
- Pacing yourself, balancing rest and exercise
- Planning and prioritizing
- Problem-solving
- Using energy-saving tips and assistive devices

THE PAIN/FATIGUE CYCLE

Tricyclic antidepressants that relax muscles and promote sleep help people with fibromyalgia break out of the chronic pain-fatigue cycle.

send the signals to your brain, where they are recognized as pain. The process stimulates the formation and release of chemicals called endorphins, which are naturally occurring painkillers.

However, researchers believe that the alarm system works differently in people with fibromyalgia. For one thing, they may have increased levels of substance P, the neurotransmitter that heightens pain perception, and lower-than-normal levels of serotonin. (See chapter 1 for more information on these substances.) These chemicals affect the pain response.

Acute pain, such as the pain of touching a hot stove, tells you that to prevent further injury you need to do something in a hurry, like move your hand away from the stove. Chronic pain, as in fibromyalgia, sends a stubborn, low-key, more general distress signal.

Although chronic pain may be telling you something's wrong, interpreting the pain is usually more difficult than interpreting acute pain. If the chronic pain is due to fibromyalgia, your body may be asking for changes such as more rest, medications, relaxation or exercise.

As one saying goes, "Pain may be inevitable, but misery is optional." No magic solution can rid you of chronic pain, but you can find ways to manage it. Your pain can be a signal for action rather than an ordeal to be endured.

The Gate Theory of Pain

Pain can vanish without apparent reason. People with severe injuries may feel nothing at first. Or pain can flare, traveling to uninjured parts of the body.

Why does this happen? One concept is the *gate theory of pain*. This theory proposes that as pain signals travel to and from the brain, they pass through a "pain gate" that can be opened or closed by various factors – which you may be able to learn to control.

Factors that can "close" or narrow the gate and block pain signals include nerve impulses and release of endorphins. Certain medicines, such as morphine and other narcotic pain relievers, imitate the body's endorphins and block the pain signal. Techniques that block or alter pain perception include stimulation of the skin in or near the area of pain with heat, cold, acupuncture, liniment or electrical stimulation such as EEG biofeedback. Similarly, positive stimuli, such as pleasant thoughts and humor, can alleviate pain by distracting you from it.

On the other hand, negative emotional experiences, such as stress, mental and physical fatigue, anxiety and depression can "open" or widen the gate and intensify pain perception. That's why your pain can seem worse if you feel depressed, tired or stressed.

Researchers believe that people with fibromyalgia process pain differently than people without the condition (see Chapter 1). One theory suggests that, over time, repeated pain stimuli causes some part of the pain system to change, a "wiring" mistake now known as *central sensitization*. As a result, the central nervous system begins to interpret what is normally not painful (for example, being touched on the shoulder) as very painful, a condition called *allodynia,* and also develops a heightened sensitivity to pain, known as *hyperalgesia.*

What doctors don't know is whether the pain of fibromyalgia causes central sensitization or vice versa. Despite these challenges, people with fibromyalgia may learn techniques to help manage this often debilitating pain.

WHAT OPENS THE PAIN GATE?

It's easy to slip into the habit of taking too much medicine or drinking too much alcohol to escape pain. These unhealthy habits may aggravate your symptoms by weakening your general health or by deepening anxiety, depression and fatigue. Although you may have some bad days when your fibromyalgia pain flares, if you answer "yes" to any of the questions below, you may choose to find healthier ways to handle pain.

• Do you use up your pain medication faster than you used to?

• Do you drink alcohol several times a day?

• Do you spend all day in bed on a regular basis?

• Do you talk about pain or fibromyalgia most of the time?

• Do you smoke to relax?

• Do you feel as though your life is one unpleasant chore?

WAYS TO CLOSE THE PAIN GATE

There are a number of safe methods that you can use to address fibromyalgia pain and narrow the pain gate. Your doctor may be

Avoid Injury or Burns

To avoid injury or burns, follow these safety tips for using heat and cold treatments:

• Use only on dry and healthy skin; the treatment could irritate a pre-existing skin condition. Dry yourself thoroughly after bathing and before using a heat treatment.

• Protect the skin over any bone that is close to the surface of your skin. Place extra padding over the area to prevent burning or freezing.

• Treat each area for only 15 to 20 minutes at a time. Let your skin return to its normal temperature before another application.

• Put a towel between your skin and any type of cold or hot pack.

• After the treatment, check the area for any swelling or discoloration.

• Gently move the painful areas to reduce stiffness.

• Do not use an electric device unless it is UL (Underwriter's Laboratory) approved and in good repair.

able to prescribe medication to help you deal with fibromyalgia pain, but you also can try any of the following methods to help you manage it.

• **Heat and cold treatments.** Apply heat or cold to a sensitive area to reduce pain and stiffness. Heat and cold are old but effective remedies. Most people find heat treatments of 20 minutes or less best before exercising. These treatments relax your muscles and stimulate circulation. These heat treatments include heating pads or warm baths. Cold packs, which seem most helpful after exercise, are especially good for acute pain, numbing the sore area and decreasing inflammation and swelling. Cold treatments include gel packs you can keep in your freezer or even bags of frozen peas. Use cold treatments for no more than 15 minutes. Follow the advice of your physician or physical therapist when using these methods, especially heat.

• **Exercise.** Another key to coping with pain is following a gentle exercise program designed by your doctor or physical therapist. A program of flexibility and endurance exercises, such as walking or water exercise classes, will help relieve stiffness and give you an improved sense of well-being. Exercise is one of the most vital elements of controlling the symptoms of fibromyalgia. (See Chapter 6 for in-depth information.)

• **Massage.** Fibromyalgia patients consistently say that massage is one of the few techniques that offer them temporary pain relief. Massage relieves muscle spasm and increases blood flow, bringing warmth to sore areas. Also, massage temporarily relieves pain and muscle tension, which can help you relax and sleep better.

If your shoulders, elbows, wrists or fingers are in pain, you may not be able to or may not want to give yourself a massage. If that's the case, ask your doctor or a reputable medical organization to recommend a professional massage therapist experienced in working with people with fibromyalgia.

If you massage your own muscles, try using an electric massage device. Some have infrared heads that direct heat to painful areas. Use lotion or oil to help your hands glide over your skin. Menthol gels also provide a comforting tingle.

Here are some tips for safe massage:

• Stop if the massage is causing you pain.

• Don't massage an area that is swollen or painful. Massage may make it worse.

• If you use a menthol gel, always remove it before using a heat treatment. Otherwise you might burn yourself.

• To find a professional massage therapist, ask your doctor, physical therapist, local hospital or medical society for a referral. If you belong to a fibromyalgia support group, ask other members if they can recommend a good massage therapist.

• Be sure any professional is licensed in massage therapy (denoted by LMT after their name) or is a physical therapist who has treated patients with fibromyalgia. Ask for a reference from a client. If the therapist says he or she can "cure" your fibromyalgia, search for another therapist.

PROPER BODY MECHANICS

Body mechanics is the positioning of the body when we stand, walk, sit or change positions. Good body mechanics – proper posture, using our stronger joints to carry loads, keeping things close to the body for leverage, not reaching or straining our lower back, shifting positions from time to time – help us perform daily activities in ways that are less aggravating to painful areas. These body mechanics tips will help reduce pain:

• **Good posture.** Good posture puts the body in the most efficient and least stressful position, protecting your neck, back, hips and knees. Slouching when driving or sitting in a chair is an example of poor posture, which can tire you and add to your pain.

• **Standing.** Use your entire body to stand correctly. Imagine a straight line connecting your ears, shoulders, hips, knees and heels. Now unlock your knees, tighten your stomach muscles and tuck your buttocks under. Hold your shoulders back, tuck your chin in a comfortable position, and stand with your feet apart and spread slightly, or with one a little in front of the other to keep your balance.

If standing for a long time becomes painful, sit down. Both of these actions flatten your back and prevent slouching.

• **Sitting.** Your spine should be stable and supported when you sit. To sit correctly, use pillows or a rolled-up towel to support your lower back. Place your hips, knees and ankles at a 90-degree angle (with a footrest, if necessary). Hold your shoulders back, and tuck your chin in a comfortable position.

Your shoulders should be relaxed with your arms at your side, elbows at a 90-degree angle or lower, and your wrists straight. You may need to use an adjustable chair to position your joints for different work surfaces, such as a desk or counter. Sit in a higher chair if it is difficult to sit down or stand up. Use a book stand to avoid neck strain when you look down to read.

• **Lying Down on Your Back.** Sleep with a small rolled towel in your pillowcase or use a cervical (or neck) pillow to avoid stressing your neck or neck muscles.

• **Lying on Your Side.** Support your arms and legs with several soft pillows or a large body pillow.

• **Lying on Your Stomach.** Lying on your stomach is acceptable for good body mechanics, as long as you are careful not to turn your neck too far toward your shoulder or overarch your back. Place a pillow under your head to help keep it turned forward, minimizing neck rotation. Put another pillow under your stomach to flatten any arch in your back.

• **Body Leverage and Load Distribution.** Hold objects close to your body when lifting or carrying. This method is less stressful. Slide objects across the floor whenever possible instead of lifting and carrying them.

Use your large, strong joints and muscles to lift or carry, and spread the load over stronger joints or larger surface areas. For example, carry a purse with a shoulder strap, bearing the weight on your larger shoulder joints to ease stress on elbows, wrists and fingers. Or use a waist pack instead of a purse to eliminate stress on your lower back and improve posture. Use your palms instead of your fingers, and your arms rather than your hands, to lift or carry items. When climbing stairs, step up with your stronger leg, and step down using your weaker leg. Always use the handrail.

• **Movement.** Staying in one position for a long time adds to stiffness and pain. Do a quick check of your jaw, neck, shoulders, arms, wrists, fingers, hips, legs, ankles and toes. Stretch and relax areas that are tired or tight.

ARTHRITIS FOUNDATION • 125

• **Weight Control.** Extra pounds add stress to hips, knees, back and feet, leading to additional muscle strain. (Having just eight extra pounds is the equivalent of carrying a gallon of milk wherever you go.) If you are overweight, check with your doctor or nutritionist for advice about a weight-loss and exercise program. You'll have more energy and feel healthier.

Energy-Saving Techniques

Plan ahead, organize and create shortcuts to save energy. By reducing your fatigue and placing less stress on tired muscles, you may also help control pain. The following lifestyle tips make sense for everyone, especially people with fibromyalgia:

• Combine errands and chores to get more done with less effort.

• Plan simple meals that require little preparation. Reheat leftovers on plates in the microwave (no pots and pans to wash). On days you can spare the time and energy, cook extra portions to freeze.

• Don't be penny-wise and pound-foolish. Is driving an extra 15 minutes to a discount store really worth saving 50 cents on light bulbs? Your time and energy are at least as valuable as gasoline. Keep shopping short and simple.

• Sit when you work. If that's not possible, take short rest breaks.

• Whenever possible, transport items on a cart to avoid carrying them.

• Use assistive devices (see box on pages 126 - 127) to reduce stress on your tired muscles. Helpful products can do the following:

• Provide leverage: Try lever faucets, tap turners, key devices and doorknob extenders.

• Extend your reach: Try long-handled items such as shoehorns, tool extensions and bath sponges.

• Save labor: Try electric can openers, pre-washed and pre-cut fresh vegetables, electric car windows and garage-door openers.

• For more practical advice on adapting activities when you have chronic pain or fatigue, look for *The Arthritis Foundation's Tips for Good Living With Arthritis,* a book of handy tips like the ones listed here. Call 800-207-8633 to order, or go to the Arthritis Foundation Web site at www.arthritis.org.

REVAMP YOUR BODY MECHANICS

Using good body mechanics – the proper alignment of your skeleton – as you go about your daily tasks can save you from pain and conserve your energy as well. Try readjusting your posture as you do the following:

• Reading: Sit in a firm chair with stable spine support instead of lying down in bed or on your side. Place your book so you don't have to look down.

• Preparing food/washing dishes: To ease the strain on your back, place one foot on a footstool and stand up straight, without leaning forward – or open a lower cabinet door and prop one foot on the cabinet ledge.

• Working at the computer: Buy a comfortable chair with good low-back support and arm rests. Position your wrists so that they are in line with your forearms. Lean forward at your hips instead of bending at the waist or neck.

- Driving: Get a car with adjustable bucket seats, arm rests and a head rest you can position to support the middle of your head. Sit up straight, keep your seat upright and don't pull your seat too close to the steering wheel. Add a back rest for support.

EMOTIONS AND COPING

Because negative emotions can make your pain worse, your attitude plays an important role in coping with illness. People with fibromyalgia who feel helpless and depressed about their condition have a tendency to decrease their activities, develop poor self-esteem and just feel generally worse. You can build a sense of control by making positive adjustments to your thoughts and actions. Thinking differently may not get rid of your pain, but having a more positive attitude can help you feel better overall.

MIND-BODY TECHNIQUES

Mind-body techniques, such as biofeedback, meditation, yoga and breathing exercises, are all relaxation techniques that can reduce the body's stress response, and improve the delivery of oxygen to the muscles and brain. Biofeedback involves working with health-care professionals to control your body responses by watching electrical monitors that record heart rate, skin temperature, brain waves and muscle tension. Meditation, yoga and breathing exercises teach ways of breathing slowly and deeply to promote muscle relaxation and stress relief. Although these methods are not cures, many studies have shown them to be effective in relieving chronic pain.

A "GOOD LIVING" LIFESTYLE

Having fibromyalgia can lead to a life built around pain and sickness. If you've been

RESOURCES FOR ASSISTIVE DEVICES

Assistive devices are products that help you perform ordinary tasks more easily with less strain on your joints and muscles. They are also called self-help aids, adapted equipment or ergonomic equipment.

The companies listed below offer assistive devices and ergonomic equipment for the office and the home. This list is by no means complete, nor is the list an endorsement by the Arthritis Foundation, but it may give you a good place to begin searching for useful products. You can request catalogs from these companies so you can order items on your own, or you can order products through a physical or occupational therapist.

Consult a physical or occupational therapist, or speak to your doctor, to find more sources of self-help or assistive devices.

DAILY LIVING EQUIPMENT

Concepts ADL
P.O. Box 339
Benton, IL 62812
800/626-3153

Human Touch Inc.
200 S. Desplaines
Chicago, IL 60661
312/258-0888

focusing on your illness, try devoting your attention to achieving good health instead. Think positively, indulge your sense of humor, enjoy a balanced diet, exercise regularly and welcome activities with others. Follow your treatment plan, take your medication, practice relaxation techniques and reach out for help when you need it, whether from a doctor, therapist or other health professional.

RELAXATION

Pain and stress have similar effects on the body. Muscles tighten and breathing becomes fast and shallow. Heart rate and blood pressure rise. Relaxation can reverse these effects. It also endows a sense of control and well-being, making pain easier to manage.

Relaxation is more than just sitting down to read or watch TV. It involves learning to calm and control your body and mind. These skills don't come easily, especially if you are in pain. Practice can help you achieve relaxation. The best time to use relaxation skills is before your pain becomes too intense. Chapter 13 offers a full explanation of different types of relaxation techniques.

DISTRACTION

Try taking your mind off pain by focusing on someone or something else. The more you concentrate on something outside your body, the less you will be aware of physical discomfort. Seek out engrossing interests – a new hobby, sport, computer game, book or movie. Or help others by volunteering in your community, such as at a church or local charitable organization.

NCM
Consumer Products Division
P.O. Box 6070
San Jose, CA 95150-6070
800/235-7054

Sears Home HealthCare
P.O. Box 19009
Provo, UT 84604
800/326-1750

Smith and Nephew
P.O. Box 1005
Germantown, WI 53022
800/558-8633
262/251-7840

ERGONOMIC OFFICE EQUIPMENT

Ergonomic Solutions
129 N. Sylvan Drive
Mundelein, IL 60060-4949
847/566-4949

Ergo Source
4250 Norex Drive
Chaska, MN 55318-4374
800/969-4374

Ergonomic Technology
135 Carlisle Road
Deerfield, IL 60015
847/945-0009

HUMOR

Can laughter be the best medicine? Medical research suggests that humor has beneficial effects on the mind and body, particularly when it comes to restoring health and fighting pain.

William F. Fry, MD, a professor of psychiatry at Stanford University Medical School whose research focuses on the physiological effects of laughter, estimates that 20 seconds of robust laughter beneficially works the heart much like three minutes of hard rowing. Laugh 100 times today, and you get the physical benefits of riding a stationary bike for 15 minutes, including a calorie-burning boost in metabolism. In fact, changes that occur during mirthful experiences involve the muscular, respiratory, cardiovascular, endocrine, immune and central nervous systems.

It's clear that for people in pain, laughter is a great distraction, has no side effects, and can even help control pain. It's not necessary to howl with laughter, according to Clifford Kuhn, MD, a professor of psychiatry at the University of Louisville School of Medicine. Even faking a smile helps your body release endorphins and give you a lift.

Try the ideas below to keep your humor quotient high:

Clear a path to good humor. Julie Kurnitz, an actress and singer in New York City who has Marfan syndrome, a genetic disorder of the connective tissues that affects the heart, joints and eyes, begins her humor workshops for health professionals and people with chronic illness by sticking prewritten Post-It notes all over her body. Each note represents one of the day's stresses. Then she plucks off the ones that no longer matter. A run in her stockings? She can buy a new pair. No hot water? She can shower at the Y. Her now-laughing class follows suit. "We're usually so cluttered with stresses, we couldn't see humor if it hit us over the head," says Kurnitz.

Look for humor in unlikely places. Look for irony or unintentional humor in newspaper advertisements or street signs. If you pass an automotive repair shop advertising a "certified mechanic on duty," remember that in England, "certified" is a slang term for "insane."

Make humor happen. Dr. Kuhn hangs cartoons on the refrigerator and buys funny ties, shirts and underwear. Kurnitz blows bubbles in her workshops and strings Christmas lights across her bookshelves. Put whatever makes you smile or laugh in plain view so you can access humor when you need it most. [Excerpted from "Comic Relief" by Dorothy Foltz-Gray, *Arthritis Today*, November/December 1998.]

ACTIVITY: Create Your Own Pain-Management Plan

Now that you've read this chapter, you have some idea of how to control pain. Consider charting your pain-control methods to keep track of which methods work best. Adapt this worksheet to your own purposes. Post it on your refrigerator or medicine cabinet where you can refer to it often. Another form of the worksheet follows on the next page.

WORKSHEET: My Pain-Management Plan

Use the following worksheet to record the strategies you plan to use for pain relief. That way you'll have a ready reference when you need it.

Medications: _____

_____

Schedule: _____

_____

Heat, cold, massage: _____

_____

Relaxation techniques: _____

_____

Exercises: _____

_____

Other techniques (distraction, humor, pleasant thoughts): _____

_____

WORKSHEET: My Pain-Management Plan

I take these medications at these times: _____

Name of medication: _____

Schedule: _____

Heat, cold, or massage can help my pain. What I will do: _____

_____

When will I do it: _____

_____

Rest is important in managing my pain. I will rest: _____

_____

Excercise can help my pain and stiffness. I will do (types of excercises): _____

_____

I will do these excercises (how often/when): _____

_____

Being calm and relaxed helps the pain. My ways to practice relaxation are: _____

_____

I will practice _____ times a day.

Keeping my mind off the pain is important. When I'm in pain, I will think about (list some pleas-

ant thoughts or memories): _____

_____

I need to focus on healthful habits. One new healthful habit I'm going to practice is:

_____

I'm going to ask my doctor or therapist these questions about my treatment program:

_____

Resources, address & phone numbers:_____

Local Arthritis Foundation chapter: _____

Local fibromyalgia organization: _____

Doctor: _____

Therapist(s): _____

Pharmacist: _____

Other members of my health-care team: _____

Chapter 11

Feeling Exhausted:

How To Cope With Fatigue

In healthy people, a few late nights or excessive physical exertion can cause fatigue, a feeling easily alleviated by a nap or a good night's sleep. But in 75 percent to 80 percent of people with fibromyalgia, fatigue is an ongoing and significant problem – an all-encompassing blanket of exhaustion.

What Is Fatigue?

Fatigue is physical and mental exhaustion. Fatigue is a state that can be caused by several factors, such as emotional stress, physical illness, poor sleeping habits, poor eating habits and depression. Fatigue often results in an impaired ability to do the normal activities of the day. You may feel listless, sleepy or unable to sustain exercise or exertion.

Fatigue may come and go, but it also may be perpetuated by the poor sleep that often accompanies fibromyalgia. Many people with fibromyalgia often wake up feeling tired, even after sleeping through the night. Although sleeplessness contributes to fatigue, so can other factors (such as those mentioned above), so getting more sleep may not relieve the fatigue associated with fibromyalgia.

Certain factors, such as sleep, that affect fatigue are addressed elsewhere in this book. Getting a good night's rest is covered in Chapter 12. Exercise, another essential treatment for restoring energy, is covered in Chapter 6. Many pain-management techniques in Chapter 10 also battle fatigue, including tips on narrowing the pain gate through proper body mechanics, energy-saving and assistive devices. On the flip side, the unhealthy habits described in Chapter 13 – smoking, drinking and negative thinking – can deepen fatigue.

Managing fatigue means walking a fine line between doing too much and doing too little. Many people with fibromyalgia push themselves so hard that they make themselves worse. Others surrender to exhaustion and

Sample Priority Sheet

Make a list of basic priority questions, and fill in your own responses to determine what activities are most vital to you.

What is most important to you?
- Cooking, spending time with my family and friends, my job.

What activities are relevant to the priorities you've identified?
- Grocery shopping, cleaning, activities with family and friends, going to work.

What must you accomplish?
- Going to work.

What can you eliminate?
- Grocery shopping and cleaning. My family can do these chores, or I can use a grocery delivery service and investigate using a cleaning service.

What can you ask other people to do?
- I don't have to cook every night. We could all take turns. And the nights I do cook, my family can clean up.

What can be modified or simplified?
- I don't have to make such ambitious meals. And maybe I could work part-time instead of full-time.

What can you say no to?
Sometimes you must say no to yourself as well as to other people.
- I can quit my volunteer jobs. And my house doesn't have to be spic and span. I can say no to perfection.

give up activity altogether. They, too, only increase their fatigue through inactivity.

This chapter is about finding a balance. You probably won't be able to eliminate fatigue completely. But you can lessen it by setting priorities and conserving your strength for whatever you value most.

Setting Priorities

To get a clearer idea of what is important to you, develop a "to-do" list that distinguishes between what you *have* to do and what you *want* to do. List everything you do during a typical week, and then rate each activity's importance. Try a simple scale of ratings: A = must be done; B = should be done; or C = would like to do. Look at your daily routine and responsibilities in light of your energy, and then ask these questions:

What is most important to you personally? Think in basic terms of family, work, friends, church or synagogue, hobbies.
- What activities are relevant to the priorities you've identified?
- What must you accomplish?
- What can you eliminate?
- What can you ask other people to do?
- What can be modified or simplified?
- What can you say no to? Sometimes you must say no to yourself as well as to other people.

PACING YOURSELF

No matter how well you prioritize, if you don't pace yourself, you may not have the stamina to carry out your plan. Estimate your energy level realistically, and allow for adjustments as your fibromyalgia worsens or improves. Here are some tips:

• Take breaks during or between tasks, before you get tired. A ratio of 10 minutes of rest to 50 minutes of activity works well for many. When your fibromyalgia is more active, rest longer and more frequently.

• Alternate light and heavy tasks, doing the toughest jobs when you're feeling best. Stick to the time you've allotted for work, and then quit. You'll get more done in the long run if you don't wear yourself out.

• Don't rush. You'll be more efficient working at a comfortable pace than at a hectic one that invites mistakes and accidents. Schedule time for the unexpected.

• Divide big jobs into little ones.

• Avoid activities that tax you beyond endurance. For some people, that might mean the New York Marathon. For others, it's attending the monster truck rally your husband insists you'll enjoy. Just say no.

Problem Solving for Fatigue

The following examples at right offer ways to solve problems that may lead to fatigue. In the example below, the problem is analyzed. Use the numbered points to apply the same logic to your situations. Ask family and friends for suggestions when you get stuck.

Plan To Act Against Fatigue

Describe one cause of your fatigue in the blank chart on p. 139, and write down

Problems and Alternatives

PROBLEM: Because of the pain and fatigue associated with your fibromyalgia, you are having difficulty maintaining your yard.

ALTERNATIVES: Consider other options that will help you achieve this task:

Change method or environment:
• Sit to do trimming.
• Use proper body mechanics.
• Hire a caretaker.
• Plan a patio garden of container plants rather than large beds.
• Move to an apartment or condominium where a groundskeeper provides lawn care.
• Work in small areas each day.
• Plant low-maintenance ground cover instead of grass.
• Have flower beds built at waist-high level to prevent stress on your back.

Use equipment:
• Use a self-propelled lawn mower or a riding mower.
• Use long-handled trimming devices and weeding tools.
• Keep a stool nearby for rest periods.

Avoid heavy lifting:
• Use a cart to move equipment.
• Use lightweight equipment.
• Ask a friend or family member to help with lifting.

options for dealing with it. Consider the advantages and disadvantages of each option, and then try one.

PROBLEM-SOLVING FOR FATIGUE

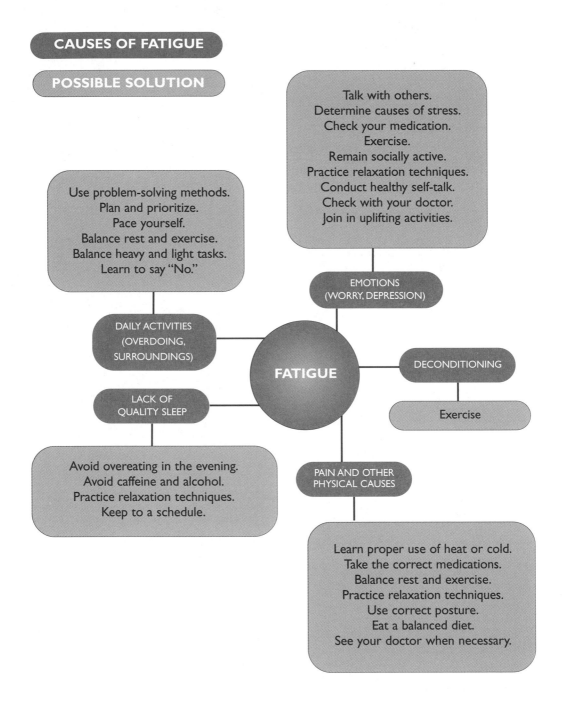

CAUSES OF FATIGUE

POSSIBLE SOLUTION

Talk with others.
Determine causes of stress.
Check your medication.
Exercise.
Remain socially active.
Practice relaxation techniques.
Conduct healthy self-talk.
Check with your doctor.
Join in uplifting activities.

Use problem-solving methods.
Plan and prioritize.
Pace yourself.
Balance rest and exercise.
Balance heavy and light tasks.
Learn to say "No."

EMOTIONS
(WORRY, DEPRESSION)

DAILY ACTIVITIES
(OVERDOING,
SURROUNDINGS)

FATIGUE

DECONDITIONING

LACK OF
QUALITY SLEEP

Exercise

Avoid overeating in the evening.
Avoid caffeine and alcohol.
Practice relaxation techniques.
Keep to a schedule.

PAIN AND OTHER
PHYSICAL CAUSES

Learn proper use of heat or cold.
Take the correct medications.
Balance rest and exercise.
Practice relaxation techniques.
Use correct posture.
Eat a balanced diet.
See your doctor when necessary.

WORKSHEET: Fatigue Problem Solving

CAUSE OF FATIGUE	POSSIBLE SOLUTIONS

Chapter 12

Resting Well:

The Keys to a Good Night's Sleep

Lack of sleep and abnormal sleep patterns are hallmarks of fibromyalgia and may be the major culprits behind your fatigue. This chapter will help you understand your sleep problems and identify ways to improve your sleep.

What Is Normal Sleep?

As essential to our bodies as breathing, sleep can be under-appreciated in a 24-hour culture. This most basic part of our daily life rhythm is vital to every dimension of health and well-being.

Scientists are just beginning to discover sleep's complexities. They've learned that sleep is not just a period of rest, but a time for critical body functions to occur, including the release of key hormones that regulate body processes such as healing and renewing tissue. Scientists also now know that the type of sleep we experience varies throughout the night and throughout our lives.

Sleep, controlled in part by the *hypothalamus*, a part of the brain that regulates many basic body functions, occurs in stages. Stage 1 is a transition between wakefulness and

sleep, lasting from about 30 seconds to several minutes. Stage 2 is the first level of true sleep. This is the stage in which sleepers spend most of their time.

In stages 1 and 2, the brain sends out alpha waves, which are fast-moving waves that measure brain activity. These two stages of sleep may be known as *alpha sleep*.

However, the deepest, most restorative sleep occurs later, in stage 3 and stage 4. In these stages, you're least likely to be awakened by an outside noise. Delta waves, or slow brain waves, occur only during this part of sleep, so stages 3 and 4 are sometimes referred to as *delta sleep*. Without delta sleep, you don't feel relaxed and refreshed in the morning.

Over the course of the night, you move in and out of sleep stages several times. If anything arouses you, you may awaken fully or partially to be in stage 1 sleep, then drift back successfully into stages 2, 3 and 4.

The stage of sleep during which you dream is known as *REM sleep,* named after the rapid eye movements that occur under closed lids during this phase. The first REM cycle of sleep occurs about 90 minutes after you fall asleep, and it lasts only five minutes. REM sleep repeats approximately every 90 minutes. In addition to dreaming, REM sleep is also when we store information in long-term memory.

The optimum amount of sleep a person needs differs with age. Although we often hear that the average person needs about eight hours of sleep each night, scientists are finding that sleep requirements are individual, determined by each person's biological clock. The need changes across your life span and with life events, such as illness or injury.

An infant needs long stretches of sleep throughout the day. A small child needs one lengthy, sustained period during the night and at least one nap during the day. An adult usually needs one sustained period that is shorter than a child needs, although studies show that even this formula varies.

Some people can adapt well to having their sleep divided into segments during the day and night, but they still need delta sleep during those separate segments. Older people tend to awaken earlier, and they awaken more easily to sound or other disturbances. But they never outgrow their need for delta sleep. They tend to make up lost sleep by drifting off during the day. Interruption or

lack of delta sleep is a key factor in fibromyalgia fatigue, as well as other symptoms. As we learned in Chapter 1, delta sleep is the time when the body secretes important hormones and regenerates energy for the rest of our day.

Fibromyalgia and Sleep

People with fibromyalgia often wake feeling that they haven't slept at all. That's because they tend to have a higher proportion of alpha-wave sleep than normal, leading to what's called *alpha-delta intrusion*. Their excess alpha waves intrude on delta, or deep, sleep, rousing them again and again during the night. Consequently, they get considerably less delta sleep than most people. Cheated of its restorative effects, people with fibromyalgia often feel fatigued and overwhelmed by the need to nap.

Factors That Can Disturb Sleep

Begin improving your sleep by eliminating factors that may contribute to sleep problems. These factors can stem from your diet, personal habits, stress or other lifestyle elements.

In order to improve sleep, first try to make your sleeping environment a restful place. Address problems of excessive heat, cold, light or noise, and make the bedroom the most comfortable haven possible. Next, examine the following factors to see if any could be interfering with your sleep.

MEDICATIONS

If used occasionally, medications such as sleeping pills can be helpful. However, if used nightly, they can produce an abnormal form of sleep, robbing you of REM sleep. Without REM sleep, you are deprived of your most important dream periods, a situation that eventually can cause you to have nightmares. Also, some sleep medications can cause side effects like next-day grogginess, especially in older people whose bodies process drugs more slowly. A medication called zolpidem tartrate (*Ambien*) may avoid this problem, as its effects last only four to six hours and do not disrupt deep sleep. Take *Ambien* only as prescribed by your doctor, who will assess its interaction with your other medications.

DRUGS AND FOODS

Many drugs can interfere with sleep. Glucocorticoids (such as prednisone), which have many uses, including the relief of allergies and joint inflammation, may cause sleep difficulties, especially if the dosage is high. Cold medicines that contain antihistamines, headache medications that contain caffeine, and antidepressants (such as *Prozac*) are other causes of sleeplessness.

Caffeine in soft drinks, coffee and tea also can cause problems. If you have trouble sleeping, try eliminating caffeine from your diet by switching to non-caffeinated beverages. There are many decaffeinated brands of coffees, teas and soft drinks. Speak to your physicians about the drugs you are taking, including over-the-counter drugs such as diet pills, that may contain caffeine. Older people, in particular, develop a progressive sensitivity to caffeine and also may find that excessive sugar can trigger sleeplessness.

EATING AND DRINKING HABITS

We are all familiar with the experience of lying awake at night after eating too much or eating the wrong kind of food. The resulting stomach distress can make sleep difficult. For example, if you are lactose-intolerant, drinking a glass of hot milk before bedtime (a common home remedy for sleeplessness) is the worst thing you can do for your sleep. Eating a spicy or greasy meal might cause indigestion that keeps you from sleeping soundly. Also, avoid drinking too much fluid before bedtime. If you have to get up in the middle of the night to urinate frequently, you may find it difficult to go back to sleep.

SMOKING

Smoking is an unhealthy, dangerous habit and it is important to quit smoking if you now smoke. Smoking is a leading cause of heart disease and several forms of cancer. Although some people say they smoke to relax, nicotine actually stimulates the nervous system, making falling asleep more difficult.

If you do smoke, ask your doctor for assistance in quitting. There are many programs and prescription treatments available to aid you in this healthy lifestyle change. Smoking among teenagers has risen in recent years, so if you are the parent of a teenager with fibromyalgia, encourage your child to quit smoking and find professional help if you need it.

DRINKING ALCOHOL

Alcohol, a depressant, can help you doze off, but you may awaken after your body processes the alcohol and have difficulty returning to a restful sleep. The psychological and physical effects of alcohol-induced depression can make fibromyalgia worse. Speak to your doctor or other health-care professional about the amount of alcohol you regularly drink, and ask if drinking may be interfering with healthy sleep.

STRESS

Stress can hamper your ability to sleep. If you have gone through an upsetting experience, or if you take the day's problems to bed, relaxing is difficult. But working long hours and then lying in bed trying to forget about the job is a common problem in our society. The problem intensifies if you use your bedroom as an office or study. Instead, try to use your bedroom for rest and relaxation only. There are many tips for relieving stress in Chapter 13.

PHYSICAL PROBLEMS

Any annoying feeling – whether it's a pain or an itch – can make it hard to sleep. People with fibromyalgia sometimes try to ignore their pain during the day, perhaps minimizing or skipping their pain medication. Then at night they find the pain impossible to ignore.

Take your medications as prescribed, even when you feel better. A dose of your pain reliever at bedtime will work much better if you listen to and take care of your body during the day, as well as at bedtime.

Hormonal fluctuations also can present challenges to sleep. Many women have trouble sleeping during their menstrual period when levels of a hormone called *progesterone* temporarily drop. Pregnancy-related hormonal changes also affect sleep patterns, especially in the first three months and in the final month of pregnancy. Also, the hot flashes and night sweats associated with menopause, when estrogen levels decline, may awaken a woman from a sound sleep or keep her from getting to sleep.

Periodic limb movement disorder (PLMD, formerly known as *nocturnal myoclonus)* is a benign type of muscle contraction that occurs as a twitch or jerk of the leg or legs at the start of sleep. Many people with fibromyalgia report having this problem. Your sleep partner may be the first to notice the problem, but in any case, it can disturb your ability to get deep sleep, whether you are aware of this or not. PLMD can be treated with a tricyclic antidepressant drug called clonazepam (*Klonopin*).

Another potential leg problem is *restless leg syndrome*. This syndrome causes peculiar sensations of crawling, spasticity, twitching or pain in the legs that provoke a need to move them. The result is repeated interruptions of sleep or an inability to fall asleep. Your physician may prescribe dopaminergic drugs such as carbidopa/levodopa (*Sinemet/Sinemet CR*), or clonazepam, which can help relieve this problem in most people.

Tips for Improving Your Sleep

- Maintain a regular daily schedule of activities, including a regular sleep schedule.

- Exercise, but not in the late evening.

- Set aside an hour before bedtime for relaxation.

- Eat a light snack before bedtime. You should not go to bed hungry, nor should you feel too full.

- Make your bedroom as quiet and as comfortable as possible. Maintain a comfortable room temperature. Invest in a comfortable mattress and/or try a body-length pillow to provide more support.

- Use your bedroom only for sleeping and for being physically close to your partner.

- Arise at close to the same time every day, even on weekends and holidays.

- Avoid caffeine (in coffee, tea, cocoa, soft drinks) and alcohol before bedtime.

- Avoid long naps. If a nap is needed to get you through the day, keep it short, and schedule it well in advance of your bedtime. Try exercising in the afternoon rather than napping.

- Avoid sleeping pills.

- Don't smoke. If you must smoke, don't smoke before bedtime.

- Use a clock radio with an automatic shutoff to play soft music at bedtime. If you are not a heavy sleeper, wake up to music rather than a clanging alarm.

- Take a warm bath before going to bed.

- Listen to soothing music or a relaxation tape.

- Read before bedtime if you like, but avoid suspenseful, action-filled novels or work-related material that can preoccupy your thoughts and cause a poor night's sleep.

- Use earplugs or white noise to block distracting noises.

- Before going to bed, write down your worries and make a "things-to-do" list. Then put it away for tomorrow so you can stop thinking about them.

- If you don't go to sleep within the first 30 minutes after going to bed, or if you wake up in the middle of the night and can't get back to sleep, get up and go to a different room. Try a relaxation technique, read, or listen to soothing music.

Some people have a condition called *obstructive sleep apnea*, a difficulty breathing when they sleep, which in turn keeps them from getting a restful night's sleep. The problem occurs when airways become blocked during sleep. Although the condition is unrelated to fibromyalgia, it obviously increases sleep difficulties. It's best to arrange for a sleep specialist to confirm the condition in a sleep laboratory. Because breathing difficulties are more common in those who are overweight, weight reduction may be a solution. Your doctor also may recommend a continuous positive airway pressure device, or CPAP, to keep airways open while you sleep.

Treatments for Sleep

There are a number of drugs, both prescription and over-the-counter, and supplements to help you alleviate the sleep problems associated with fibromyalgia.

Tricyclic antidepressants or benzodiazepines such as zolpidem (*Ambien*), florazepam (*Dolmane*), tenazepam (*Restoril*), oxazepam (*Serax*), quazepan (*Doral*), and estazolam (*ProSom*) may be helpful. Antihistamines, used for allergy relief, cause drowsiness, including diphenydramine (*Benadryl, Tylenol PM, Sleep-eze*), dimenhydrinate (*Dramamine*) and meclizine (*Bonine*).

Many people who have problems sleeping choose to purchase over-the-counter supplements at pharmacies and health-food stores instead of getting a prescribed drug from their doctors. Two common supplements used as sleep aids are *melatonin* and *valerian root*. As with any herbal remedy, take melatonin or valerian root only on the advice of your physician.

Melatonin, a hormone made by the pineal gland in the brain, helps regulate sleep. Available in pill or capsule form at health-food and supplement stores, a 3- to 6-mg. dose works as a sleep aid for four to six hours. Melatonin's effectiveness as a sleep aid has received a great deal of media attention recently. In a 1999 study at the Medical College of Wisconsin in Milwaukee, people with fibromyalgia who took melatonin for six months slept better the first month but in subsequent months showed no difference from those taking a placebo. In fact, those taking melatonin had a higher level of anxiety. Also, a small amount may cause a large increase in the body's melatonin, and the long-term effects of this are unknown.

Valerian root's effectiveness was the subject of a 1998 German study, in which researchers found that the root of this wildflower works as well as *Librium*, a tricyclic antidepressant, to help sleep difficulties, minus any addictive effects. Valerian root is taken in capsule form or as a tincture.

Part Five

Master Emotional Challenges

Chapter 13

Achieving Relaxation:

How To Master Stress

Stress — even from small, everyday hassles like snarled traffic, long grocery lines, missed buses, sick kids or a busy phone signal — can cause damage to the health and well-being of a person with fibromyalgia. Minor stresses can be more detrimental in their constancy than major stresses, such as moving to a new house. Having a chronic health condition like fibromyalgia can add a new set of challenges and daily adjustments that only increase a person's susceptibility to stress.

What Is Stress?

By definition, *stress* is the body's physical, mental and chemical reaction to frightening, exciting, dangerous or irritating circumstances. Too much stress can exacerbate fibromyalgia symptoms. For instance, part of our response to stress is to breathe faster and less deeply. That change puts the body on alert, tensing the muscles, which in turn increases muscle pain. Stress also weakens the immune system, leaving you more vulnerable to other illnesses, and it also can add to anxiety, depression and poor sleep.

Still, stress is an inevitable part of living. A move to a new town, a change in jobs, divorce or the death of someone close to you — all these situations can be stressful. Not all stressful events are unpleasant or negative. Planning a wedding or getting the family ready for a summer vacation can also be nerve-racking.

Now that you have been diagnosed with fibromyalgia, you may have to rely upon family members and health-care professionals more than in the past. You may have to alter your lifestyle or give up favorite activities because of limited abilities. None of these changes is easy, and all can be upsetting. By learning to understand and manage your stress, however, the adjustments will be easier to handle. You can reduce your pain, feel healthier and manage your condition more effectively.

Healthy vs. Unhealthy Stress

Stress is supposed to be a temporary response, an emergency setting that revs our engines and shifts us into high gear. But if you get stuck on that setting, stress becomes unhealthy. This section outlines some differences between healthy and unhealthy stress.

Healthy stress is followed by relaxation. Your life has demands, but it also should have resources that help you rebound from stress. A stressful job may be a demand that causes stress, but your ability to put your aggravation behind you when you leave work should be a resource. After you've dealt with the situation, your body returns to its pre-stressed state: Heartbeat and breathing slows, blood pressure goes down and muscles relax. Your physical and emotional energies recharge, so that you can meet the next challenge.

Unhealthy stress occurs when demands exceed your resources. You have a stressful day at work but cannot put the stressful events behind you when you leave work. You stay geared up, and you don't relax. Your body is still in a stressed state: heart racing, blood pressure up, muscles tight, palms sweaty, stomach knotted. Because you aren't relaxing, your body and mind are unable to recover energy and balance, so the

Effects of Chronic Stress

• Headaches
• Stomach distress, ulcers
• High blood pressure
• Muscle tension, back pain and other types of pain
• Chronic fatigue
• Restlessness, irritability, frustration
• Decreased zest for life, worry, fear, depression
• Difficulty making decisions, forgetfulness
• Increased use of alcohol, cigarettes or drugs
• Eating and sleeping problems
• Disease flares
• Poorer immune function

next challenge is difficult to meet. With each challenge, your physical and emotional resources become more exhausted. The stress has become chronic. Chronic stress can cause many negative effects on your body and mind, summarized in the table at right.

How Your Body Reacts to Stress

When you feel stressed, your body becomes tense, and the muscle tension can increase your pain. Increased pain can make you feel helpless and frustrated by limiting your abilities, which in turn can lead to depression. If you understand how your body reacts to stress physically and emotionally, and you learn how to manage stress, you can help break the destructive cycle.

PHYSICAL CHANGES

At times, you may feel unable to deal with stress in a positive way. In other words, you cannot let go of stress and this tense state becomes constant. With no outlet, constant stress takes its toll on your body. Tension can lead to headaches, upset stomach or worsened fibromyalgia symptoms. Research shows that stress also may affect the body's immune system, leading to illness, fatigue or other physical problems.

Research also suggests that fibromyalgia patients may respond to stress differently than other people, producing less of a hormone called *corticotropin-releasing hormone* (*CRH*). CRH normally helps signal the body to release stress hormones, including adrena-

Listening to Your Body

Be aware of stress signals:
1. Headaches
2. Stomach upset
3. Emotional reactions
4. Sleeping problems
5. Other signs

Some warning symptoms
1. Tight shoulder, arm or neck muscles
   Hunched shoulders
   Clenched teeth

2. Stomach knot or butterflies
   Stomachache
   Appetite loss
   Diarrhea or constipation

3. Anxiety
   Moodiness
   Anger
   Hopelessness
   Low self-esteem
   Poor concentration
   Depression

4. Trouble falling asleep
   Waking up early, being unable to fall asleep again
   Oversleeping, sleeping too much
   Disturbing dreams

5. Chronic fatigue
   Cold, clammy hands
   Heart pounding
   Chest feels tight or heavy
   Dry mouth

line, to help the body deal with an emergency. But too little CRH may lead to lowered amounts of adrenaline, which puts the body in a chronic state of perpetual stress and contributes to an overall ill feeling. Chapter 1 has more information on hormones and their connection to fibromyalgia's symptoms and possible causes.

EMOTIONAL CHANGES

Your mind's reaction to stress is harder to predict than your physical reaction to it. Emotional reactions vary, depending on the situation and the person. They may include feelings of anger, fear, anxiety, helplessness, loss of control, annoyance or frustration. A small amount of stress actually can help people perform their best in high-pressure situations, such as competing in an athletic event or performing on stage. Under too much stress, however, people may become accident-prone, commit errors and perform clumsily.

Each person responds to stress differently. You may like to be busy, or you may prefer a slow pace with less activity. What you find relaxing may be stressful to someone else.

Problem Solving for Stress

The key to managing stress is to make it work *for* you instead of *against* you. Consider the following steps for managing your stress:
1. Recognize your body's stress signals.
2. Identify what causes your stress.
3. Change what you can to reduce stress.
4. Manage or accept what you can't change.
5. Adopt a lifestyle that resists stress.

RECOGNIZE YOUR BODY'S STRESS SIGNALS

Each of us responds to stress differently, physically and emotionally. One person's stress shows up as headaches and tight shoulder muscles. Another person may seldom get headaches, but always gets an upset stomach.

Stress symptoms often are obvious, but not always. For example, a stress headache may begin as a slightly aching neck that you ignore until it turns into a pounding pain.

Sample Stress Diary

DATE	CAUSE OF STRESS	TIME	PHYSICAL SYMPTOMS	EMOTIONAL SYMPTOMS
4/18	getting kids off to school	7 a.m.	fast heartbeat, tightness of neck	feel rushed, disorganized
4/18	stuck in traffic	8:30 a.m.	headache, heart beating faster, legs aching	frustrated, angry at being late
4/18	meeting presentation	10 a.m.	fast heartbeat, dry throat, clammy palms	anxious, nervous

WORSHEET: Keeping a Stress Diary

Record the events in your life that cause stress, as well as any physical or emotional symptoms that result. After one week, look for patterns in symptoms, determine what causes them and make life adjustments.

DATE	CAUSE OF STRESS	TIME	PHYSICAL SYMPTOMS	EMOTIONAL SYMPTOMS

Or you may assume that a digestive upset was caused by something you ate – until you notice the same thing happens every time you confront a stressful situation. By listening to your body, you can learn how stress affects you personally.

IDENTIFY WHAT CAUSES YOUR STRESS

What causes you the most worry and concern? What situations leave you anxious, nervous or afraid?

Learning what causes stress is a personal discovery. The things that may cause you stress, whether it's car trouble, a long line at the bank or an overcooked roast beef, may not bother someone else. Once you know what the stressful aspects of your life are, you can decide how to change them or adapt to them.

CHANGE WHAT YOU CAN TO REDUCE STRESS

Once you've identified the causes of your stress, determine which stressful situations can be changed, and change what you can control. Here are some strategies:

• **Set goals.** Develop a plan for achieving goals, one that includes hobbies and friends, and that delegates responsibilities. And be flexible about the time your goal will take to achieve.

Reality Check

Learn to put stressful situations in perspective by asking these questions:

• Does this situation reflect a threat by signaling harm or a challenge by signaling an opportunity?

• Are there other ways to look at this situation?

• What exactly is at stake?

• What is the worst that can happen?

• What are you afraid will occur?

• What evidence do you have that this will happen?

• Is there evidence that contradicts this conclusion?

• What coping resources are available?

• **List your priorities.** What needs to be done immediately? What can be done later? What can be eliminated? You may need to buy groceries today, but perhaps you can wash the clothes tomorrow.

• **Eliminate daily hassles.** If rush-hour commuting bothers you, map out a new, more peaceful way to work. Scale back your work hours; it's likely that the company will survive. Avoid annoying people and places. If you have to see them, decide not to let them get on your nerves. Use the Hassles Scale on page 154 in this chapter to identify stressful situations in your life.

• **Let uplifting activities outnumber hassles.** Use the Uplifts Scale on page 153 to rate your progress in incorporating uplifting activities into your life.

• **Pamper yourself.** Ask: "Does this decision or action take care of, or work for, me?" It's easy to take care of others at the expense of your own health. Take time do things you enjoy.

• **Plan for special events.** Then you can enjoy them rather than collapse from stress. Shop early or year-round for holidays or birthday gifts so you won't be caught in a last-minute crush. Buy many cards at once – for birthdays, weddings, new babies and anniversaries – and store them, so you won't have to shop for each occasion. If you're entertaining, choose easy-to-prepare foods and buy the rest. Or make it a potluck bash.

• **Acknowledge major life events as stress sources.** Even positive events like graduating from school, finding a new job or taking a vacation can be stressful. Try to recognize the important changes in your life so that you

Uplifts Scale

Uplifts are events that make you feel good. They are sources of your contentment, satisfaction and joy. Put a check by any events that may have made you feel good in the last <u>month.</u> **Optional:** Rate how <u>strongly</u> you feel that each of the following uplifts improves your spirits on a scale of 1 to 3 (1 = somewhat strongly; 2 = moderately strongly and 3 = extremely strongly). Then add up your total score. Compare to the score on your Hassles Scale on the next page. Aim for getting an Uplifts score that is at least twice your total Hassles score.

	✔		✔
1. Getting enough sleep		23. Spending time with friends	
2. Being lucky		24. Buying things for yourself or home	
3. Saving money		25. Home pleasing you	
4. Not working		26. Giving or getting a present	
5. Having a pleasant conversation		27. Traveling	
6. Feeling healthy		28. Doing yardwork	
7. Being pregnant		29. Making a friend	
8. Visiting, phoning or writing someone		30. Getting unexpected money	
9. Relating well with your spouse or lover		31. Dreaming	
10. Completing a task		32. Pets	
11. Being efficient; meeting responsibilities		33. Children's accomplishments	
12. Cutting down on smoking		34. Things going well at work	
13. Cutting down on drinking		35. Making decisions	
14. Losing weight		36. Confronting someone	
15. Good sex		37. Being alone	
16. Friendly neighbors		38. Knowing your job is secure	
17. Eating out		39. Feeling safe in your neighborhood	
18. Using drugs or alcohol		40. Fixing something	
19. Having plenty of energy		41. Meeting a challenge	
20. Relaxing		42. Flirting	
21. Having the "right" amount of things to do		Other uplifts, not mentioned yet:	
22. Good times with friends		43.	

Hassles Scale

Hassles are irritations that can range from minor annoyances to fairly major pressures. Listed here are a number of ways in which a person can feel hassled. Go through the list and put a check by those hassles that have happened to you in the past month. **Optional:** Rate how severe each hassle has been on a scale of 1-3 (1 = somewhat severe; 2 = moderately severe; and 3 = extremely severe). Then, add up your total score. Compare the score on your Uplifts Scale (see previous page). Aim for getting an Uplifts score that is at least twice your total Hassles score.

	✓			✓
1. Misplacing things		23. Not getting enough sleep		
2. Trouble with neighbors		24. Problems with your children		
3. Social obligations		25. Problems with your parents		
4. Health of family member		26. Problems with your spouse or lover		
5. Concerns about debts		27. Too much to do		
6. Smoking too much		28. Work unchallenging		
7. Drinking too much		29. Legal problems		
8. Trouble relaxing		30. Concerns about weight		
9. Trouble making decisions		31. Not enough enengy		
10. Problems with people at work		32. Feeling conflict over what to do		
11. Customers/clients giving you a hard time		33. Not enough time for family		
12. Home maintenance		34. Property, investments, taxes		
13. Concerns about job security		35. Yardwork		
14. Don't like current job		36. Concerns about news		
15. Bored		37. Crime		
16. Lonely		38. Traffic		
17. Fear of confrontation		39. Pollution		
18. Illness		Other hassles not mentioned yet:		
19. Physical appearance		40.		
20. Problems at work		41.		
21. Car trouble		42.		
22. Rising prices		43.		

can prepare for them and better understand your emotional and physical reactions.

- **Learn to say no.** And lose the guilt. It's OK to let other parents chaperone the zoo trip. Turning down extra duties even temporarily can reduce your stress.
- **Think "win/win."** When resolving conflicts, seek solutions that will benefit both sides. If you want to go for a walk, and your spouse has chores to do, help finish the work and go walking together.

MANAGE OR ACCEPT WHAT YOU CAN'T CHANGE

You can change only yourself, not other people. Some situations can't be changed, but your point of view can. Try to roll with the punches. Being flexible helps you keep a positive attitude, despite hardships. Here are some ways to help you change your outlook.

- **Think positively.** Ask yourself if there is any hidden benefit to the stressful situation, and make the most of it. Getting fired or laid off from a job could lead to a spiral of depression, debts and debilitating pain. Or it could be the opportunity you've been looking for to change your work situation for the better.
- **Run a reality check.** Try to evaluate the situation's real importance. Your daughter didn't call this week. Does this omission mean she's ignoring you, or that her own schedule was difficult to manage? And will your world collapse because she didn't call?
- **Develop and use support systems.** Share your thoughts with family, friends, clergy or others who are good listeners. Such

sharing may help you see problems in a constructive way. However, don't whine to others constantly about every detail of your discomfort. You may alienate your support structure and isolate yourself from the help you need, and you may be reinforcing your own bad habit of focusing on your pain.

- **Refocus your attention positively.** Thinking about something or someone else besides yourself can help you relax and distract you from pain.
- **Develop safety valves.** Release stress through healthy, productive methods such as exercising or writing your thoughts in a journal.
- **Have fun.** Schedule time for leisure activities that lighten your spirits. Join others for activities that make you laugh and distract you from your stress and pain.

ADOPT A LIFESTYLE THAT RESISTS STRESS

Learning how to relax is one of the most important ways to cope with stress. Relaxation is more than just sitting back and being quiet. It is an active process to calm your body and mind, and this process requires practice. Once you know how to relax, it becomes second nature. As you learn new methods, keep these principles in mind:

- Stress has many causes, and it has many solutions. The better you understand what causes your stress, the more successfully you can manage it.
- Not all relaxation techniques work for everyone. Try different methods until you find one or two that you like best. You may

learn that some techniques work well for certain situations, while others work better at other times.

• Learning these new skills takes time. Practice new techniques for at least two weeks before you decide if they are working.

If you need help learning how to relax, see a mental-health professional or contact your local Arthritis Foundation chapter. You can locate your nearest chapter by calling 800/283-7800, or visit the Foundation Web site, www.arthritis.org.

A few common techniques for relaxing are described below, as well as several relaxation activities. See the Resources section of this book for more information on ways to manage the stress of fibromyalgia.

RELAXATION TIPS

Use the following techniques to relax your body and mind.

• Pick a quiet place and time when no one will disturb you for at least 15 minutes.

• Make yourself as comfortable as possible. Loosen any tight clothing and uncross your legs, ankles and arms. Sit in a comfortable chair or lie down.

• Try to relax daily or at least four times a week.

• Don't expect immediate results. It may be several weeks before you reap benefits.

Relaxation should be enjoyable. If these techniques are unpleasant or make you more nervous and anxious, stop. You may be able to manage your stress better with other techniques.

JOIN A SUPPORT GROUP

Support groups don't have to be, and shouldn't be, pity parties where participants swap stories of woe. To feel the empathy of peers is great, but to feel positive thoughts replace negative ones is also wonderful. Below are a few types of groups you can join that could energize your way of thinking.

• **Cognitive behavioral therapy.** This type of therapy involves education, stress-reduction techniques, family support and exercises designed to change negative ways of thinking and behaving. For example, a person who constantly apologizes for his behavior may practice praising his behavior instead. Studies show that such therapy can be beneficial for those with fibromyalgia.

• **Yoga.** Yoga is a form of mental, spiritual and non-impact physical exercises originated in ancient India. The exercises involve gentle stretches and deep breathing that improve flexibility and relaxation, reduce anxiety and increase body awareness.

• **Meditation.** Meditation is another ancient practice that involves deep breathing and a single focus on a word, object, thought or sensation. Research suggests that meditation can lower blood pressure, heart rate and stress levels.

Activity: Deep Breathing

Deep breathing is a basic technique that applies to almost all relaxation exercises. This simple technique is a key to mastering the art of unwinding. Here are the steps:

1. Get as comfortable as you can. Loosen

any tight clothing or jewelry, uncross your legs and arms, and close your eyes.

2. Place your hands firmly but comfortably on your stomach. This will help you feel when you are breathing properly. When you breathe correctly, your stomach expands as you breathe in and it contracts when you breathe out. (Many people breathe "backwards"; they tighten their stomachs when they breathe in, and relax their stomachs when they breathe out. If you breathe backwards, take a minute to get your motions coordinated.)

3. Inhale slowly and deeply through your nose to a count of three. Feel your stomach push against your hands. Let it expand as much as possible as you fill your lungs with air.

4. When your lungs are full, purse your lips (as if you were going to whistle) and exhale slowly through your mouth for a count of six. (Pursing your lips allows you to control how slowly or quickly you exhale.) Feel your stomach shrink away from your hands.

5. When your lungs feel empty, close your mouth and begin the inhale/exhale cycle again.

6. Repeat the inhale/exhale cycle three or four times at each session.

7. Whenever you're ready, slowly open your eyes and stretch.

Tip: Breathing deeply can make you feel light-headed or dizzy, especially if you are tired or hungry. At first, it's a good idea to practice deep breathing while you are sitting or lying down. Once you get the hang of it, deep breathing can be done anytime, anywhere.

Activity: Relaxation to Control Pain

Preparation: First, take time to make sure that you are in a comfortable position. Check from head to toe to determine whether your whole body is being supported. Adjust any parts that feel uncomfortable. Try not to have legs or arms crossed, but above all, do what is comfortable for you.

Now, close your eyes. Become aware of your breathing. Feel the movement of your body as you breathe in and out. Breathe in slowly and exhale. On your next breath, focus on an image of breathing in good, clean air and exhaling all your tensions with your breath out. Slow your breathing and focus on releasing tension each time you breathe out.

MIDDLE PART:

Option 1: *"Pain Drain"* Now, feel within your body, and note where you experience pain or tension. Imagine that the pain or tension is turning into a liquid substance. The heavy liquid flows down through your body and out through your fingers and toes. Allow the pain to drain from your body in a steady flow. Now, imagine that a gentle rain flows down over your head and further dissolves the pain into a liquid that drains away. Enjoy the sense of comfort and well-being that follows.

Option 2: *"Disappearing Pain"* Now, notice any tension or pain that you are experiencing. Imagine that the pain takes the form of an object or several objects. It can be fruit, pebbles, crystals or anything that comes to mind. Pick up each piece of pain, one at a time, and place it into a magic box.

As you drop each piece into the box, it dissolves into nothingness. Now, again survey within your body to see if any pieces remain and remove them. Imagine that your body is lighter now, and allow yourself to experience a feeling of comfort and well-being. Enjoy the feeling of tranquility and repose.

Option 3: *"Healing Potion"* Now, imagine you are in a drugstore stocked with bottles and jars of exotic potions. Each potion has a special magical quality. Some are pure, white light, others are lotions, balms and creams, and yet others contain healing vibrations. As you survey the potions, choose one that appeals to you. It may even have your name on the container. Open the container and cover your body with that magical potion. As you apply it, let any pain or tension melt away, leaving you with a feeling of comfort and well-being. Imagine that you place the container in a special spot and that it continually renews its contents for future use.

Option 4: *"Leaving Pain Behind"* Imagine that you are dreaming. Although your body will stay in the same position, imagine that you are leaving it. As you leave, notice that you have left your tension and pain behind. Pick a special spot to visit, one that brings pleasure and a feeling of well-

being. Notice how your dreamlike body feels as you visit this special place. Linger here for a while and when you feel ready, return to your body. When you open your eyes, retain the freedom from tension and pain, and continue to experience a sense of comfort and well-being.

END PART:

Whenever you are ready, slowly stretch and open your eyes.

Adapted from The ROM Dance, a range-of-motion and relaxation program by Diane Harlowe and Patricia Yu, 1992. Materials available from The ROM Dance, P.O. Box 3332, Madison, WI 53703 or by calling 800/488-4940.

GUIDED IMAGERY

Think of guided imagery as a daydream with a tour guide. By diverting your attention away from stress, guided imagery takes your mind on a mini-vacation. Use your imagination to transport yourself to a more peaceful place. For some people the most relaxing place is the seashore; for others it's the mountains. Pick your mind's ideal vacation spot, and go there.

Activity: Guided Imagery Smorgasbord

The following exercise teaches you how to focus on relaxing in your choice of desirable, stress-free locations. Have a friend read the exercise to you, or record it yourself, and play it back as you imagine.

BEGINNING RITUAL:

Get as comfortable as you can, feet slightly apart, arms resting at your sides. Now close your eyes. Take a slow, deep breath through your nose and slowly exhale through your mouth. Again, take a deep breath and slowly exhale. Continue to breathe slowly and deeply. Notice yourself getting more and more relaxed. Let all your tension melt away.

MIDDLE PART:

Option 1: *"Sea"* Your body is very heavy, at ease and warm. Listen to your heart beating steadily and regularly. As you listen to your heart, you feel its beat in your whole body. It feels as though you are on a boat on a quiet, calm sea with the water lapping against the sides.

You're inhaling and exhaling in time with the waves. They are gently rocking you. The rocking continues in your mind and as you rock, negative emotions are dropping out of you one after the other – frustration, sorrow, depression, heartache, worries, resentment. You feel serene and content.

You feel so wonderful, you'd like the whole world to enjoy it with you. Out of the depths of your heart rises a great lightness, and you feel it flow in a continuous steady stream through your whole body, and all the time you feel lighter and lighter.

Adapted from the Arthritis Movement Workshop Leader's Manual, Arthritis Foundation, Arizona Chapter.

Option 2: *"Pine Forest"* Imagine that you are sitting comfortably in a chair or hammock in the middle of a pine forest. You can smell the cool, clean, fragrant air. You breathe deeply and feel the gentle, cool breeze on your skin.

You feel peaceful and calm. As you look around, you are impressed by the beauty of the tall pine trees with their rich, brown bark and graceful, feathery branches. You notice the pinecones. You watch the leaves of the aspen trees rustle in the wind. You study the ground, with its rich, brown dirt covered with pine needles and leaves, its robust, earthy aroma.

You hear birds, a woodpecker at work in the distance. You notice a small clearing in the forest covered with green grass and wildflowers. You are at peace in the pine forest, relaxed and calm.

Adapted from the Systemic Lupus Erythematosus Self-Help Course Leader's Guide by Katalina McGlone, 1984.

Option 3: *"Ocean Beach"* Imagine that you are at the ocean. You are sitting comfortably on the beach under the shade of a large beach umbrella. Feel the warm sand, the comfortable air around you, and the refreshing, soft breeze blowing through your hair. Feel the warm moisture in the air upon your face. Notice the smell of the ocean. Imagine how beautiful, how brilliantly blue the sky is.

You're sitting on the beach feeling calm, peaceful, relaxed, comfortable. You are watching the waves as they grow and break, mesmerized as they go in and out from the shore. You can hear the thundering of the waves as they break. The only other sounds are those of the seagulls.

Notice how peaceful you feel sitting on the beach feeling in harmony with nature.

Adapted from the Systemic Lupus Erythematosus Self-Help Course Leader's Manual, Katalina McGlone, 1984.

Option 4: *"Memory and Fantasy"* In this relaxation exercise, remember a past experience – or create a new one – with your imagination.

Imagine yourself in an environment where you feel secure, comfortable and relaxed. This can be a place you remember, a fantasy you are creating, or a mixture of memory and imagination. Simply experience whatever comes to you. Sometimes the environment will change during the exercise, and sometimes it will remain the same.

Place yourself in this environment and note how you are positioned: standing, sitting, or lying down. In this secure, comfortable, relaxed environment, look around you. Take in the panorama of colors, forms and textures. If you are outside or can see outside, note the season, the time of day or night, the weather. Look all around you: in front, behind, to both sides, above and below you. Look at the sky or ceiling, the ground or floor in the distance and up close. Are there other people here? Take in all you wish to see. What sounds come to you? Listen for sounds in the distance, up close, all around you. From what directions do the sounds come?

In this secure, relaxed and comfortable environment, is there anything that you can smell? If something to drink or eat presents itself, taste it fully and note its texture in your mouth. Is there anything or anybody you are touching? How does it feel? How does the environment around you feel physically: warm or cool, damp or dry? Do you feel movement in the air? How does it feel

emotionally? How do you feel inside in this environment?

Once again, take in the sights around you. They may have changed. Note the sounds, smells, tastes and sights. Focus on emotional feelings – the feelings inside.

Adapted from The ROM Dance, a range-of-motion and relaxation program by Diane Harlowe and Patricia Yu, 1992. Materials available from The ROM Dance, 408 South Baldwin Street, Madison, WI 53703, or by calling 800/488-4940.

Option 6: *"Water Fantasy"* Imagine that you are immersed in water, perhaps in your bathtub, in a lake, a swimming pool or even a whirlpool bath. Imagine that the water is the perfect temperature, just warm enough so that every muscle in your body feels as supple and flowing as the water itself. Experience the water flowing around and coming into contact with each part of you. As it does this, it melts away deeper levels of tension, leaving your body feeling cleansed and drained of tension.

Let yourself stay in this wonderful water for a while, all the time continuing to allow yourself to let go of deeper and deeper levels of tension, allowing yourself to feel more and more relaxed.

.Adapted from The ROM Dance.

END PART:

You may go back to this place whenever you want by sitting quietly and remembering this place in as much detail as possible. Whenever you are ready, move your fingers, wiggle your toes, and come back to this world feeling refreshed and invigorated.

BUILD UP YOUR RESISTANCE TO STRESS

Stress can have a negative effect on your body. Taking good care of your body can help you build up resistance to stress. Ways to take good care of your body include:

- eating a balanced diet
- exercising
- avoiding drugs and alcohol
- getting enough rest and sleep
- saving energy by pacing your activities
- accentuating the positive

Incorporate the relaxation techniques you've learned in this chapter into your daily life and you'll reap rewards. Managing your stress – whether or not you have fibromyalgia – can lessen pain and increase good living.

Chapter 14

Losses and Gains:

Getting Past Grief and Depression

Chronic illness may change your life in so many ways that you'll sometimes wonder if you're the same person. It's not surprising that after the initial relief of diagnosis, when you have a name for your problem at last, grief sets in. Yet this pervasive feeling of loss catches many people with fibromyalgia by surprise.

What Is Grief?

Grief is a natural response to loss. Usually, we think of grief in terms of death or divorce. Feelings of grief over the diagnosis of a chronic illness are not discussed very often, but chronic illness, too, involves loss.

For people with fibromyalgia, the losses are physical, social and personal. Mourning these losses is not only natural, but necessary as part of a healing process that allows you to accept the changes fibromyalgia has brought.

Giving yourself permission to grieve for your old life will help you reach acceptance sooner and put you on the path to building a new life. Your spouse and family members also may need to grieve the changes in your health. Allow them to do it in their own way and time.

A NOTE ON GRIEF AND DEPRESSION

Mental and emotional health play leading roles in the battle against fibromyalgia, more so than in many other physical conditions. Studies show that approximately 25 percent of people with fibromyalgia are clinically depressed, requiring the care of a mental-health professional such as a psychiatrist or psychologist (see Chapter 4). No one knows if depression is a cause or effect of the disorder, but depression can be overcome. Although taking command of your life and health care is difficult when you're already feeling overwhelmed and defeated, it's a must if you are to feel better.

If you've recently been diagnosed with fibromyalgia, you may be grieving the loss of the life you had before symptoms set in.

Possible Grief Responses

- SHOCK AND DENIAL: "NO! IT CAN'T BE TRUE!" Denial is a protective buffer, allowing you to replace anxious thoughts with more hopeful ones. Denial buys time for you to mobilize other coping techniques and face your losses at a manageable pace. This stage is usually temporary, but if you can't accept your diagnosis, you won't be able to fight your condition.

- BARGAINING: "LET'S MAKE A DEAL." You may find yourself making secret promises, for example, "I'll become a better person" if fate or a higher power sends a cure. Or you may begin an endless cycle of seeking other medical opinions and trying unproven remedies. This process is yet another "time-buying" stage before acceptance.

- ANGER: "WHY ME?" Anger, rage, envy and resentment are all common responses to bad news like a diagnosis of fibromyalgia. You may express your anger by criticizing your doctor, family or friends. You may put off necessary chores or treatments, or sink into depression. You may feel cheated by fate or a higher power. But if you don't move beyond this stage, you can become extremely irritable and quarrelsome.

- GUILT: "I DESERVED IT." Next, you may blame yourself for having fibromyalgia. ("I should have been a better person; I should have taken better care of myself," and so on). You may begin to think of yourself as a burden to others. And just as you view your illness as a personal failure, you think if you try harder to do more, you'll feel better.

- SADNESS AND DEPRESSION: "I WILL MISS BEING ABLE TO . . ." This stage is a natural part of saying goodbye to lost roles and abilities. It usually gets better in time. However, if this stage persists, depression will set in as a lingering sense of despair and worthlessness. It can also be a quiet cover for anger, anxiety or guilt. Depression persists until negative thinking is changed.

- FEAR AND UNCERTAINTY: "WHAT ELSE WILL HAPPEN?" Also natural responses to fibromyalgia's unpredictable variations, fear and uncertainty themselves may cause muscle tension, increased heart rate, stomach distress, and trembling. Signs that you're stuck in this stage include anticipating the future with fear and anxiety, worrying about the next bad bout even during periods of good health, or feeling helpless or out of control over your health from day to day.

- LONELINESS AND ISOLATION: "NO ONE UNDERSTANDS." Curtailing your activities can lead to fewer social contacts. Also, some friends may withdraw because they don't know how to help. Family members may become emotionally exhausted. All these factors can lead to isolation and loneliness if you don't work at broadening your support system and maintaining contact with the outside world.

- RECONCILIATION AND ACCEPTANCE: "I MAY HAVE FIBROMYALGIA BUT. . ." Acceptance is the final stage of grief, but the first sign you're ready to build a new life. Once you are able to let go of the past and the person you were before you developed fibromyalgia, you can get on with your recovery.

That's natural when you're faced with a chronically painful condition for which there is no cure. Talking to friends and family may help. But if you find you're depressed and crying frequently for more than two weeks, see a doctor. Other signs that you may need professional help for depression include thoughts of hurting yourself or others, or persistent, unshakable feelings of worthlessness. See "Depression: A Self-Test" later in this chapter.

If your depression isn't severe, you may be able to improve your emotional state by teaching that little voice in your head some new lines. Tips on breaking the habit of seeing things in black or white, of generalizing, or of viewing insignificant events as catastrophes are discussed below.

Don't allow negative thinking or depression to bar the way to feeling better. As the best manager of your condition, be ready to take on the challenges of the future.

Grief's Parade of Emotions

Grief is a process made up of many feelings, a sort of parade of emotions. In her landmark book *On Death and Dying*, psychiatrist Elisabeth Kübler-Ross, MD, described the stages of grief that terminally ill people go through, and her description has been widely applied to mourning other losses as well. (See the sidebar, "Possible Grief Responses," on the previous page.)

However, the stages of grief rarely start at one point and proceed in an orderly way to the ultimate goal of acceptance. For most people,

the grief process is more chaotic. You may not experience all the emotions, nor are you likely to experience them step by step. Your reactions may skip around, backtrack or surge together.

Grieving is a personal process that each person goes through at his or her own pace. How you move through the stages of grief depends on your support systems and your basic personality. For example, if you have always been an outgoing person with a sunny disposition, you may not experience the anger or isolation that a more introverted person may feel.

You also need to understand that grief can be ongoing. A worsening of your symptoms, the anniversary of a negative event, or the reminder of an activity that you can no longer do can provoke an unexpected reaction of grief.

DEALING WITH GRIEF AND LOSS

As you consider your losses, use the following tips to help you work through your feelings.

• **Permit yourself to experience your feelings.** Face your loss. Let yourself grieve, cry and be sad. Don't try to ignore anger or punish yourself for feeling it. These emotions are a normal part of the grieving process. As long as they don't last too long, they can help you become more comfortable with the changes in your life. However, if severe depression and crying continue for more than two weeks, see a doctor.

• **Find out what triggers your fears and emotions.** What led to your feelings? What do you need right now that you don't have?

If you know you get depressed around certain times of the year, such as an anniversary date, plan to take special care of yourself during that time or plan a special treat for yourself. Avoid situations that create anxiety. This process includes limiting the amount of time you spend around people who make you feel uncomfortable.

• **Express your fears and feelings and then let them go.** Repressing your feelings can be a form of denial, or it can stem from a fear of alienating friends and family. Repressed feelings can fester and grow. Bottling up anger, for example, can result in excessive irritability, bitterness and quarreling. Repressed feelings also can come out in other destructive ways, such as skipping your prescribed treatment. Some constructive ways of expressing your feelings include talking with others, writing in a journal, crying, screaming in the shower or pounding pillows.

• **Search for meaning.** Draw strength from your spiritual beliefs. Also, think about what positive things have occurred as a result of your fibromyalgia that might not have happened otherwise. For example you may have:

• reassessed priorities
• discovered inner strengths
• developed new hobbies
• discovered new talents
• made new friends
• increased your understanding of yourself
• increased your understanding of God, a higher power or spirituality, or
• increased your understanding of others with disabilities.

Seek professional help when and if you need it. Often, just talking with an understanding person will be enough to help you through depression or grief. But if you have trouble maintaining your daily activities, feel helpless or hopeless, or have thoughts of hurting yourself or others, seek the guidance of a mental-health professional. See the end of this chapter for help on finding referrals.

Self-Talk

Self-talk is when you converse with a voice in your head, and this discussion colors your world view and shapes your expectations. When self-talk is healthy, the voice is a cheering section urging you forward. When it's unhealthy, self-talk holds you back and makes you feel cynical about your life.

Unhealthy self-talk arises from responding automatically to situations with repetitive, negative thinking patterns. These patterns may include a tendency to generalize, to see things in terms of right or wrong and good or bad, to see manageable problems as catastrophes, to place undue significance on only one aspect of an event and to jump to conclusions. Your self-talk is unhealthy when you get stuck on thinking only negative thoughts.

Watch for signs that you may be thinking negatively. Note the way you categorize yourself or others, and the way you judge, label or condemn yourself or others. For example, you may catch yourself saying, "I can't believe what a dumb thing I did," or, "I hate the way I look today." More positive self-talk responses would be "I guess I made a mistake," or "I think I should comb my hair so I will look my best."

Note how often you use words and phrases like *can't, won't, impossible, always, never, should, ought to, must, yes, but* and *if only*. If you constantly use negative terms like these, you may be engaging in unhealthy thinking.

Following are some examples of this negative approach to life.

10 UNHEALTHY WAYS TO THINK

1. **Seeing all or nothing:** You place people or situations in black and white categories, with no shades of gray. If your performance falls short of perfect, you see yourself as a total failure.
   Healthy response: You recognize an error but place it in the context of all the things you did right.

2. **Generalizing:** You see a single, unpleasant event as a never-ending pattern of defeat.
   Healthy response: You see a single, unpleasant event as a bump in the road.

3. **Using mental filters:** You pick out a single, unpleasant detail and dwell on it exclusively so that your vision of reality becomes darkened, like the drop of ink that discolors the entire beaker of water.

WORKSHEET: Losses and Discovery List

Use the blanks below to list the losses you've experienced as a result of fibromyalgia. In the space provided, list the positive things that you may have discovered as a result.

Examples:
Loss: I have lost my independence.
Discovery: I have learned to be comfortable letting other people help.

Loss: I no longer sleep through the night.
Discovery: I feel healthier when I don't drink or eat anything with caffeine. I hardly miss it.

Loss: _____

_____

Discovery: _____

_____

Loss: _____

_____

Discovery: _____

_____

Loss: _____

_____

Discovery: _____

_____

Healthy Response: You pick out the most pleasing detail and dwell on it.

4. **Disqualifying the healthy.** You reject healthy experiences, such as an acquaintance's remark that you have a great sense of humor, by insisting that it isn't true. In this way you maintain an unhealthy belief such as, "People don't like me," which is contradicted by your everyday experiences.
Healthy Response: You embrace healthy experiences such as hearing a compliment about your sense of humor.

5. **Jumping to conclusions:** You make an unhealthy interpretation even though there are no facts that support your conclusion. Some examples:
   a. *Mind reading:* You conclude that someone is reacting negatively to you and don't find out if you are correct.
   b. *Fortune telling:* You anticipate that things will turn out badly, and you feel convinced that your prediction is an already-established fact.
   Healthy Response: You assume things are going well (that people like you, that you're doing a good job, etc.) until you learn differently.

6. **Magnifying or minimizing:** You exaggerate the importance of insignificant events (such as your mistake or someone else's achievement), or you inappropriately shrink the magnitude of significant events until they appear tiny (your own desirable qualities or another person's imperfections). This procedure is also called the "binocular trick."

Healthy Response: You celebrate your own and others' achievements, small and large. If you feel jealous, you acknowledge that and then remind yourself of your own gifts, and share others' happiness.

7. **Basing facts on your emotions:** You assume that your unhealthy emotions reflect the way things really are: "I feel it, therefore it must be true."
Healthy Response: You remind yourself that most days you feel better than you do today.

8. **Using "should" statements:** You try to motivate yourself with *shoulds* and *shouldn'ts*, as if you have to be punished before you can do anything. ("I really should exercise. I shouldn't be so lazy.") *Musts* and *oughts* are also offenders. The emotional consequence is guilt. When you direct *should* statements toward others, you feel anger, frustration and resentment.
Healthy Response: You motivate yourself by remembering the good feelings or events that come with the activity. ("Exercise is hard but, boy, I feel good afterward.")

9. **Labeling and mislabeling:** These are extreme forms of generalizing. Instead of describing your error, you attach an unhealthy label to yourself. You say, "I'm a loser." When someone else's behavior rubs you the wrong way, you attach an unhealthy label to him, such as "He's a real louse." Mislabeling involves describing an event with language that is highly colored and emotionally loaded. Example: Instead of saying someone drops off her

Personally Speaking   Stories from real people with fibromyalgia

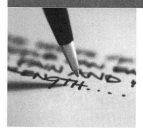

"**G**rieving the losses in chronic illness has its own peculiar difficulties. You may be struggling with your own grief while also dealing with the mourning of your family. The first time Mother came to visit after my diagnosis, she embraced me and whispered, "Here's some of your grandmother's jewelry. You might as well have it now," and "I'm glad the boys are as old as they are." I ran in stark terror.

Grief and Chronic Illness
Kathleen Lewis, RN
Decatur, GA

"However, the source of the grief process, you, is still present. You are a constant reminder to yourself and others around you of what's been lost.

"After reacting to a diagnosis of chronic illness, your family faces a period of redefinition. In this process, the family's worldview is examined and reformulated. In much the same way that you need to synthesize and incorporate a new identity, the family unit needs to also adopt one that accepts and understands your new circumstances.

"During this family redefinition, some members' roles will change. You may have always been responsible, for example, for hosting big family get-togethers, where you cooked all your specialties, polished the silverware and made sure the entire house gleamed. Now others must help – or even replace – you. In my own family, my roles as chief cook and bottlewasher at home, caretaker of my mother and source of a second income came to a crashing halt as I began to live my life from the bed to the couch to the hospital and back again. Major turmoil erupted.

"When it became clear I was seriously ill, everybody in my family pitched in – at first. Later, we hired a maid service to come in once a month to do the heavy house cleaning. The first day the maids came was like a funeral for me, even though I never relished doing housework.

"The process of renegotiating and reformulating your new family image is a major transition. Your children or spouse may resent having extra responsibilities. You may resent losing them, along with the identity those responsibilities gave you, as 'provider' or 'homemaker' or 'problem-solver.' But you may find that being 'husband' or 'mother' or 'lover' does not necessarily depend on such abilities as bringing home a fat paycheck or making the perfect puff pastry.

"Life is a highway, and you'll need to pay some tolls. If you try to run them, the consequences could be far more expensive than if you'd thrown your quarters in the basket when you came to it. In the same way, if you try to put off grief, you may well end up paying a higher price than if you face it."

From *Celebrate Life: New Attitudes for Living with Chronic Illness* by Kathleen Lewis, RN
To order this book, call 800-207-8633, or log on to www.arthritis.org.

Sample Thoughts Diary

To appreciate the power of your self-talk and the part it plays in your emotional life, make your own thoughts diary. Make a notation each time you experience an unpleasant emotion. Include everything you tell yourself to keep the emotion going.

DATE	UNPLEASANT EMOTION	SITUATION	SELF-TALK	RATIONAL RESPONSE
AUGUST 3 9:30 a.m.	depressed, frustrated	In kitchen looking at mess.	I'll never get this kitchen clean.	I'll just do a little bit and get started. No reason to do it all today.
AUGUST 4 10:15 a.m.	tired, discouraged	Putting dishes away.	I should have done a better job of straightening up.	Nothing in the world is perfect, but the room looks better.
AUGUST 6 1:00 p.m.	frustrated	Phone rings and wakes me up from nap.	I should have taken the phone off the hook.	Most days I remember to take the phone off the hook.
AUGUST 7 3:00 p.m.	depressed	Expected call from friend - it didn't come.	I have no real friends. She should have called by now.	Who says she "should" have called me? I think I'll call her.

children at day care every day, you might say she "abandons her children and lets strangers look after them."

Healthy Response: Acknowledge your error, put it in perspective, and move on. ("I'm late to the meeting. That rarely happens. I'll be on time next time.")

10. **Personalizing:** You see yourself as the cause of some unhealthy external event which in fact you were not responsible for. ("We were late to the dinner party and caused the hostess to overcook the meal. If I had only pushed my husband to leave on time, this wouldn't have happened.")

Healthy Response: You do not take on the blame that belongs to other people. ("My husband wouldn't stop watching the basketball game on TV and this made us late to the dinner party. Hey, my husband was rude, but this wasn't my fault.")

CHANGING UNHEALTHY SELF-TALK

Unhealthy self-talk can make the challenges of fibromyalgia seem like an uphill, impossible battle. Learning to change your self-talk is an important tool in reducing your stress and improving your mood. Here are some ways to make this transformation:

Unhealthy: "I would like to exercise, but I can't. I know if I did any exercise my fibromyalgia would act up. I am also too old to start exercising. I know I can't do it."

Healthy: "Starting an exercise program will give me a chance to get out of the house. I could start slow and easy with a walk in the park or the mall. If I get tired, I can sit down and look at store windows and rest for a while." Or: "Starting an exercise program will be a challenge, but I can take it slowly, and it will give me a chance to explore new types of movement."

Unhealthy: "My life will never be the same now that I have fibromyalgia. I will never be able to do anything that I like to do."

Healthy: "I'm still the same person I've always been. I can cope." Or "I've changed since I was diagnosed with fibromyalgia, but I'm still a person of worth. I still have a lot to give to people around me."

Unhealthy: "My friends never call me. People don't like being around me."

Healthy: "My friends are just trying to be considerate and spare my energy. They are waiting for signals from me. I'll call today." Or: "My friends are uncomfortable, at a loss, and don't know how to help me. I must ask them for what I need."

Activity: Keep a Thoughts Diary

Paying attention to your thoughts and feelings is the first step in gaining control of unpleasant emotions. During times of emotional turmoil, your thoughts may be so fragmented and jumbled that it's hard to know exactly what they are. Writing in a journal or in a thoughts diary is an excellent way to explore your thoughts and feelings (see the Sample Thoughts Diary on page 172). Because it's your private document, a diary can be a good safety valve for dealing with emotions and stress.

A diary or journal also can flag unhealthy thinking, serve as a reality check and help you process your feelings and thoughts. After you've been writing down your thoughts for a few weeks or months, look back at some of your earlier entries. You may find your perspective has changed. See Chapter 9 for more information on self-management.

Avoiding a Spiral Into Depression

Reactions like anger, fear and anxiety are normal parts of the grieving process. They are signals from the body and mind that all is not well and that it is time to mobilize your coping responses. When these emotions are processed by a healthy grieving person, they provide an opportunity to grow and gain new insights. But if they are not dealt with appropriately, they can cause long-term depression. The goal is to process and listen to your feelings, and then release them.

HOW TO KNOW IF YOU'RE DEPRESSED

Depression has become a catch-all term. The word sometimes is used inappropriately

Getting Self-Talk To Work for You

- Write down self-defeating thoughts.
- Do a "Reality Check." Ask:
  - Are there other ways of looking at this situation?
  - What am I afraid will occur?
  - How do I know that this outcome will indeed happen?
  - What evidence do I have that this outcome will happen?
  - Is there evidence that contradicts this conclusion?
  - What coping resources are available?
  - Have I only had failures in the past, or were there times I did okay?
  - There are times when I don't do as well as I would like, but other times I do, so what are the differences between those times?
- Change self-defeating thoughts to helpful self-talk.
- Mentally rehearse healthy self-talk.
- Practice healthy self-talk in real situations.
- Be patient – it takes time for new patterns of thinking to become automatic.

to refer to brief feelings of sadness or dissatisfaction, what we often call "the blues."

Experiencing a few depressive symptoms every now and then is part of life. But clinical, or major, depression alters the way you view the world and yourself, and may involve changes in the neurotransmitters, or chemicals, in your brain. It may last only several weeks or much longer. It may interfere with your ability to take pleasure in life, disrupt sleep and cause you to feel helpless and hopeless. Depression also can mask other emotions that are painful to face, like anger or guilt.

It can be hard to recognize depression when you're in the middle of it. Because it can come on gradually, depression can take hold of you before you realize what has happened. Look at the following chart of symptoms to help you determine whether or not you may be experiencing depression.

Remember that fibromyalgia and some of the medications used to treat it can cause some of the symptoms listed on this chart, particularly low energy and fatigue, changes in appetite and weight, and sleeping too much or too little. So these symptoms alone may not indicate depression. However, you should seek professional help if you have four or more additional symptoms that last for more than two weeks and are severe enough to disrupt your daily life.

If you ever have thoughts of death or suicide, seek professional help *immediately*. Such thoughts should never be written off as "the blues." Don't let your sad mood become a tragedy. Remember, even the most severe depression is treatable.

Activity: Depression: A Self-Test

Experiencing one or more of these depressive symptoms every now and then is a normal part of life. If a certain number of these symptoms have been bothering you for weeks or years, you may have a depressive disorder and should consult your doctor with this list in hand. See the results below.

Group 1:

Are you experiencing at least one of the following nearly every day?:

apathy, or loss of interest in things you used to enjoy, including sex sadness, blues or irritability

Group 2:

In addition, are you experiencing any of the following symptoms?:

feeling slowed down or restless

feeling worthless or guilty

changes in appetite or a substantial weight loss or gain

problems concentrating, thinking, remembering or making decisions

trouble falling asleep or sleeping too much

loss of energy, feeling tired all the time

Group 3:

And what about the following symptoms? These symptoms are not used to diagnose depressive disorders, but often occur with them.

headaches*

other aches and pains *

digestive problems*

sexual problems*

feeling pessimistic or hopeless

being anxious or worried

low self-esteem

Results:

If you have several symptoms, talk to your physician. You may be clinically depressed if you experience at least one of the symptoms in Group 1 and at least four of the symptoms in Group 2 nearly every day for at least two weeks.

Depression Risk Factors

People are at higher risk for depression at certain times in their lives or under certain conditions. You may be at greater risk if:

- You've had a previous episode of depression

- Your previous depressive episode occurred before age 40

- You have a medical condition

- You've just given birth

- You have little or no social support

- You've recently experienced a stressful life event (positive or negative)

- You abuse alcohol or drugs

- You have a family history of depression-related disorders

- You experienced only partial relief from a previous episode of depression.

Adapted from Arthritis Today Magazine

You may have chronic depression if you experience at least one of the symptoms in Group 1 and at least two of the symptoms in Group 2 nearly every day for at least two years.

*These are potential indications of depression only if not caused by another disease or by medication.

Reprinted from Arthritis Today, January/February 1996.

Seeking Professional Help

If you determine that you are clinically depressed, help is available. Seeing a mental-health professional may have once carried a stigma, but this situation is no longer the case. It's now widely recognized that seeing a therapist for help in sorting out feelings is no different from seeing a dentist for a cavity or a doctor for an infection. A psychiatrist or psychologist (for the distinctions, see Chapter 4) can help you work through your thoughts and emotions by providing an objective, listening ear and offering insight into what you may be feeling or thinking.

Newly developed medications such as SSRIs can address the imbalance of neurotransmitters, or brain chemicals, that may accompany depression. Keep in mind that a psychiatrist is the only mental-health professional who can prescribe medications, although any therapist can refer you to a psychiatrist if medications are necessary.

Even if you're not clinically depressed, you can still benefit from therapy. Dealing with the pain, fatigue and lifestyle changes imposed by fibromyalgia can be an enormous psychological challenge. Mental or emotional patterns that caused minor trouble in your life previously may now cause major problems. Relationships that functioned satisfactorily without the stress of illness may now call for restructuring and improved communication skills. Or, you may simply need a safe place to discuss your feelings. For any of these reasons, therapy might be valuable. You deserve the help you need or want.

Once you have made the decision to seek help from a therapist, how do you go about finding a qualified therapist in your area? If you have health insurance, start by getting a list of therapists your insurance provider will cover. Take this list with you as you ask around for references. Your physician may have some good suggestions. A trustworthy friend or relative who has been pleased with the services of a mental-health professional may be able to recommend someone. Another way to find a qualified therapist is to call a reputable hospital or mental-health agency in your area.

Shop around to find a qualified person who makes you feel comfortable. You will discuss personal, emotional and even intimate issues with this person, so you should feel at ease communicating your feelings with any therapist you choose.

Today, any number of people call themselves therapists although they have no licenses or training. There is nothing illegal about this practice, and some of them may be good at what they do. But your best bet is to make sure that the person you choose has appropriate mental-health education and training, and belongs to the recognized professional organization for his or her license (for example, the National Association of Social Workers). Often, such an organization will have its own telephone referral line, which will be listed in the telephone directory.

The therapist you find may be a board-certified psychiatrist, licensed clinical psychologist, licensed clinical social worker or licensed marriage, family and child counselor. Therapists who are not medical doctors, and who thus cannot prescribe drugs, may refer you for psychiatric consultation to evaluate your need for medication. See Chapter 4 for more information about different types of doctors and therapists.

Once you have obtained some names, don't hesitate to interview a prospective therapist on the phone. Ask about the person's qualifications, training and specific areas of expertise. Ask how much experience the doctor or therapist has had in treating depression. Some therapists have experience treating people with fibromyalgia, and it is perfectly appropriate to ask them if they do.

Ask about the fee for services, and make sure you know up front what your insurance will and will not cover. Do you have to pay the fee and wait for full or partial reimbursement from your insurer? You have a right to

Where To Find Help

The following organizations offer general information on depressive disorders, mental illness, and finding a therapist. Some organizations also have a referral service to help you find a credentialed therapist in your area.

American Association for Marriage and Family Therapy, 1133 15th St., NW, Suite 300, Washington, DC 20005; 800/374-2638.

American Psychiatric Association, Department AT, 1400 K St., NW, Washington, DC 20002; 202/682-6220.

American Psychological Association, 750 First St., NE, Washington, DC 20002; 800/374-3120.

Depression Awareness, Recognition and Treatment (D/ART), a program of the National Institute of Mental Health, 5600 Fischers La., Room 10-85, Rockville, MD 20857; 800/421-4211.

National Alliance for the Mentally Ill, 200 N. Blebe Rd., Suite 1015, Arlington, VA 22203-3754; 800/950-6264.

National Association of Social Workers, 750 First St., NE, Suite 700, Washington, DC 20002; 202/408-8600.

National Depressive and Manic Depressive Association, 730 N. Franklin, Suite 501, Chicago, IL 60610; 800/82N-DMDA or 800/826-3632.

National Foundation for Depressive Illness, P.O. Box 2257, New York, NY 10116; 800/248-4344.

National Mental Health Association, 1021 Prince St., Alexandria, VA 22314-2971; 800/969-6642.

Reprinted from Arthritis Today, January/February 1996.

this information, and a competent professional will not be offended by your questions.

Some therapists are willing to meet with you for an initial session without charge or at a reduced charge, so that you can make an in-person evaluation. Ask the therapist if a free initial consultation is possible.

If you don't have health insurance or if your policy doesn't cover this type of therapy, don't let that stop you from seeking the help you need. Ask your doctor to refer you to community mental-health agencies, which usually use a sliding-fee scale, based on the patient's income, family size and other considerations. Some professionals also may lower their fees, depending on a patient's financial need. And many churches, synagogues and other religious-based institutions offer regular counseling services from clergy who have additional training in therapy or counseling. For information about how and where to find reliable and affordable services, check with your local health or social-services departments.

Personally Speaking   Stories from real people with fibromyalgia

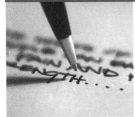

"If I could help just one person deal with fibromyalgia in a positive way, then all of my suffering has not been in vain. I truly am happy for all I have experienced. For without fibromyalgia, I would not have been able to see all that I was missing, and the necessary changes that were meant to be made in my life.

Thank God for Fibro
Marianne Vennitti
Haddonfield, NJ

"I have learned more about life, people and myself than I could ever have imagined. Now, I realize that I have so much to be thankful for. I feel as though I am one of the lucky people in this world because I was given the opportunity to stop dead in my tracks and re-evaluate who I am, what my life is all about and where I want to go for the rest of my life. I was taken off the vicious merry-go-round and placed in a protective cocoon. Within my cocoon, a transformation happened. I have grown into a much healthier and simpler human being, in mind and in spirit. I realized that all things have a purpose – something positive generates from all things that are negative.

"Within the comfort of this quiet darkness, I began to listen, hear and respond to the meaning and purpose of my life. Like a snake shedding its skin, I am working to shed all that I no longer need in my life and all the parts of my life and myself that drained me of my energy."

A Final Word

Now that you've finished this book, you have the tools to live better with fibromyalgia. As a final note, let's review the key steps to good living with fibromyalgia and how they can help you.

- **Understand fibromyalgia.** Knowledge is power, so learn as much as you can about how fibromyalgia affects your body and how it can be treated. Keep yourself informed about the latest research and treatments for fibromyalgia by reading and researching on your own.
- **Become a self-manager.** Become involved in your own health care. Do whatever you can to control the aspects of the disease that you can influence. Follow your prescribed treatment plan, and take part in monitoring your progress.
- **Adopt a wellness lifestyle.** Take steps to live a healthy life in general. Wellness practices include taking care of your body and your mind, and having a positive outlook toward life. Incorporating wellness practices into your daily life can help you feel better, too.
- **Exercise.** Exercise is a very important part of your fibromyalgia treatment plan. It is one of the most effective ways for you to reduce pain and protect your joints by strengthening the muscles around them. Develop an exercise program you enjoy and can maintain.
- **Maintain a healthy weight.** Along with exercising, keeping your weight down is one of the best things you can do for your pain. If you're overweight, take steps to gradually lose weight by modifying your diet and stepping up your exercise program to prevent further stress and muscle pain.
- **Manage pain.** This book has offered you a number of strategies for managing the pain of fibromyalgia. Some may work better than others for you, or may be better for certain situations. Experiment with these strategies, and create a pain-management plan that works for you. Then use those techniques to keep your pain at bay.
- **Handle stress and emotional challenges.** Chronic illness can bring a number of changes to your life that can affect you emotionally. Learn to take control of these emotional challenges by managing stress effectively. Seek help if the emotional aspect of chronic illness becomes more serious than you can handle alone.

GLOSSARY

acetaminophen: A type of pain reliever that does not contain aspirin and is available without a prescription under a variety of brand names.

acupressure: Application of pressure to specific muscle sites to relieve pain and muscle spasm.

acupuncture: A centuries-old method of pain relief used in China and introduced into America in recent years. Needles are used to puncture the body at sites associated with pain blockage.

acute pain: See *pain*.

adrenal glands: Glands located near the kidneys. These glands secrete *adrenaline*, a hormone that increases the heart and respiration rate when we feel frightened, threatened, or angry, preparing us to flee to safety, or stand and fight. In people with fibromyalgia, this hormone is secreted abnormally. See also *hormones*.

adrenaline: See *adrenal glands*.

aerobic: An activity designed to increase oxygen consumption by the body, such as aerobic exercise or aerobic breathing.

alpha wave: A type of electrical wave produced by the brain during quiet wakefulness. Disturbance in the production of these and delta waves, which occur during deep sleep, is characteristic of the disturbed sleep common in fibromyalgia.

American College of Rheumatology (ACR): An organization that provides a professional, educational and research forum for rheumatologists across the country. Among its functions is helping determine what symptoms and signs define the various types of rheumatic disease diagnoses and what the appropriate treatments are for those diagnoses.

antidepressants: Medications used to relieve depression or sad moods. Tricyclic antidepressants, which may relieve nighttime muscle spasms in people with fibromyalgia, work by increasing certain hormones that influence mood. A newer class of antidepressants, selective serotonin reuptake inhibitors (SSRIs) such as *Prozac*, increase the level of serotonin, a neurotransmitter that affects mood and appetite and aids sleep. Ironically, however, SSRIs may disturb sleep.

antihistamine: A drug that counteracts the action of histamine, a chemical produced in immune response (for example, when you have an allergic reaction to pollen). Histamine has powerful effects such as dilating blood vessels (thus lowering blood pressure) and stimulating secretion of gastric juices. Antihistamines sometimes cause drowsiness, a problem for people with fibromyalgia who also battle fatigue.

anxiety: A state of being apprehensive, worried or concerned.

apnea: See *sleep apnea*.

arthralgia: Pain in the joints in the absence of arthritis.

arthritis: From the Greek word "arth" meaning "joint," and the suffix "itis" meaning "inflammation." It generally means involvement of a joint from any cause, such as infection, trauma or inflammation.

autoimmune disorder: An illness in which the body's immune system mistakenly attacks and damages tissues of the body. There are many types of autoimmune disorders, including arthritis and the rheumatic diseases.

biofeedback: a procedure that uses electrical equipment to increase your awareness of your body's reaction to stress and pain and to help you learn how to control your body's physical reactions. The equipment monitors your heart rate, blood pressure, skin temperature and muscle tension. These body signals are shown on a screen or gauge so you can see how your body is reacting.

body leverage: Use of body weight, muscle strength and joints to perform any physical task, such as lifting, pulling or standing. Adapting ways of using body leverage increases efficiency and reduces muscle strain and pain.

body mechanics: The structures and methods with which your body moves and performs physical tasks.

bursa: A small sac located between a tendon and a bone. The bursae (plural for bursa) reduce friction and provide lubrication. See also *bursitis*.

bursitis: Inflammation of a bursa (see *bursa* above), which can occur when the joint has been overused or when the joint has become deformed by arthritis. Bursitis makes it painful to move or put pressure on the affected joint.

capsaicin: A chemical contained in some hot peppers. Capsaicin gives these peppers their "burn" and has painkilling properties. It is available in nonprescription creams that can be rubbed on the skin over a joint to relieve pain.

chronic fatigue syndrome (CFS): A condition manifested by long-term fatigue. The symptoms of CFS and fibromyalgia are similar, but people with CFS don't experience the pain that is characteristic of fibromyalgia.

chronic pain: See *pain*.

chronobiology: Study of the timing, rhythm, and cycles of biological events such as ovulation, secretion of hormones or temperature fluctuations.

circadian rhythm: The daily, monthly and seasonal schedules on which living things carry out essential biological tasks, such as eating, digesting, eliminating, growing and resting. Disruption of these rhythms – when you travel rapidly across time zones (promoting jet lag), for example – has a negative and sometimes profound impact on performance and mood.

continuous positive airway pressure: See *CPAP*.

control group: A group of people used as a standard for comparison in scientific studies. For example, a scientist who wants to know if daytime sleepiness is linked with fibromyalgia might study the amount of sleepiness experienced during a year in two groups: women with fibromyalgia (the study group) and women without fibromyalgia (the control group).

cool-down exercises: A series of physical activities that allow your heart and respiration rates to return to normal after being elevated by exercise.

cortisone: A hormone produced by the cortex of the adrenal gland. Cortisone has potent anti-inflammatory effects but can also have side effects.

costochondritis: Tenderness or pain in the tissue covering the rib cage and under the breasts. May be a feature of fibromyalgia.

CPAP: Stands for continuous positive airway pressure, a method of keeping the nasal airway open in people who experience chronic breathing obstruction during sleep.

deconditioning: Loss of muscle mass and strength because of inactivity. See also *reconditioning*.

deep breathing: Drawing air into the lungs, filling them as much as possible, and then exhaling slowly. Performing this type of breathing rhythmically for a few minutes increases the amount of oxygen refreshing your brain and produces relaxation and readiness for mental tasks.

delta sleep: Deep, restorative sleep; a period of sleep in which a unique type of brain wave, called the delta wave, is produced by the brain. Certain vital body functions occur during delta sleep. Disturbances of delta sleep are common in fibromyalgia.

delta wave: A type of brain wave produced during deep sleep. See also *delta sleep*.

depression: A state of mind characterized by gloominess, dejection or sadness.

disease: Sickness. Some physicians use this term only for conditions in which a structural or functional change in tissues or organs has been identified.

disorder: An ailment; an abnormal health condition.

distraction: To shift your attention deliberately from a distressing experience or sensation and focus on a pleasant or neutral one, for the purpose of relieving anxiety, stress or pain. For example, if you have fibromyalgia pain, you might focus on a favorite piece of art, music or happy remembrance instead of the pain.

double-blind studies: A method used in scientific studies to compare one intervention (such as a new medication) with other interventions or no intervention. In this method, the study participants and the persons evaluating the interventions are "blinded"– that is, they aren't told who is getting the intervention being tested – so their responses will not be influenced by their opinions or expectations of the intervention.

electrical stimulation: see *biofeedback* and *TENS*.

endorphins: Natural painkillers produced by the human nervous system that have qualities similar to opiate drugs. Endorphins are released during exercise and laughter.

endurance exercises: Exercises such as swimming, walking and cycling that use the large muscles of the body and are dependent on increasing the amount of oxygen that reaches the muscles. These exercises strengthen muscles and increase and maintain physical fitness.

ergonomics: The study of human capabilities and limitations in relation to the work system, machine or task, as well as the study of the physical, psychological and social environment of the worker. Also known as "human engineering."

exercise physiologists: Health professionals who apply their knowledge of basic physical and chemical processes in the human body to evaluate the effects and benefits of exercise. An exercise physiologist is qualified to develop individualized programs of exercise for people with fibromyalgia, arthritis and other rheumatic diseases.

fatigue: A general worn-down feeling of no energy. Fatigue can be caused by excessive physical, mental or emotional exertion, by lack of sleep and by inflammation or disease.

fibromyalgia: A noninfectious rheumatic condition affecting the body's soft tissue. Characterized by muscle pain, fatigue and nonrestorative sleep, fibromyalgia produces no abnormal X-ray or laboratory findings. It is often associated with headaches and irritable bowel syndrome.

fibrositis: An out-of-date name for fibromyalgia. Since the "itis" part of this term denotes inflammation, which is absent in fibromyalgia, physicians have dropped the term "fibrositis."

flare: A term used to describe times when the disease or condition is at its worst.

flexibility exercises: Muscle stretches and other activities designed to maintain flexibility and to prevent stiffness or shortening of ligaments and tendons.

Food Guide Pyramid: An illustration developed by the U.S. Department of Agriculture to represent the types and proportions of foods that are needed each day for a healthy diet.

Food Labeling Act: Recent legal decree of the U.S. government mandating the type of information that must be given on food labels regarding nutritional content. This Act ensures that consumers will have easy-to-read fat, protein, fiber, carbohydrate and calorie content information and more.

gate theory: A theory of how pain signals travel to the brain. According to this theory, pain signals must pass a "pain gate" that can be opened or closed by various positive (e.g., feelings of happiness) or negative (e.g., feelings of sadness) factors.

genetic predisposition: Susceptibility to a specific disease or illness caused by certain inherited characteristics.

glucocorticoids: A hormone produced in your body and related to cortisone. Glucocorticoids can also be synthetically produced (that is, made in a laboratory) and have powerful anti-inflammatory effects. These are not the same as the dangerous performance-enhancing drugs that some athletes use to promote strength and endurance.

good posture: The most efficient and least stressful body position for standing, walking, sitting, working and reclining.

grief: Feelings of loss; acute sorrow.

guided imagery: A method of managing pain and stress. Following the voice of a "guide," an audiotape or videotape, or one's own internal voice, attention is focused on a series of images that lead one's mind away from the stressor or pain.

hormones: Concentrated chemical substances produced in the glands or organs that have specific – and usually multiple – regulatory effects to carry out in the body. See also adrenaline, hypothyroidism, neural hormones, pituitary (gland), serotonin, steroids.

hypothalamic-pituitary-adrenal (HPA) axis: One of the main brain-hormonal stress response axes (i.e., places where brain function and hormonal function are coordinated in response to stress).

hypothalamus: A portion of the brain, buried deep within the skull, that has a regulatory role in many of your body's most vital functions, including progression through the stages of sleep.

ICF-1: See *somatomedin C*.

illness: Poor health; sickness.

immune response: Activation of the body's immune system.

immune system: Your body's complex bio-chemical system for defending itself against bacteria, viruses, wounds and other injuries. Among the many components of the system are a variety of cells (such as T cells), organs (such as the lymph glands) and chemicals (such as histamine and prostaglandins).

inflammation: A response to injury or infec-tion that involves a sequence of biochemi-cal reactions. Inflammation can be general-ized, causing fatigue, fever and pain, or tenderness all over the body. It can also be localized, for example, in joints, where it causes redness, warmth, swelling and pain. Inflammation is not a symptom of fibromyalgia.

internist: A physician who specializes in inter-nal medicine, sometimes called a primary-care physician.

interstitial cystitis: A chronic inflammatory condition affecting the bladder wall. Symptoms included pain in the bladder and pelvic region, urinary urgency and fre-quency. The disorder affects about ten per-cent of people with fibromyalgia.

irritable bowel syndrome: A chronic, nonin-flammatory disease that gives no clues, such as changes in cell structure, about its cause. Symptoms include abdominal pain, painless diarrhea, constipation and some-times alternating bouts of diarrhea and constipation.

isometric exercises: Exercises that build the muscles around joints by tightening the muscles without moving the joints.

isotonic exercises: Exercises that strengthen muscles by moving the joints.

juvenile primary fibromyalgia syndrome: Fibromyalgia in children.

lactose intolerance: Inability to digest lactose, which is contained in milk.

lupus (systemic lupus erythematosus): The term used to describe an inflammatory connec-tive tissue autoimmune disease that can involve the skin, joints, kidneys, blood and other organs and is associated with antinu-clear antibodies.

massage: A technique of applying pressure, friction or vibration to the muscles, by hand or using a massage appliance, to stimulate circulation and produce relax-ation and pain relief.

massage therapist: One who has completed a program of study and is licensed to per-form massage.

meditation: A sustained period of deep inward thought, reflection and openness to inspiration.

metabolism: Your body's continuous chemical and physical processes, consisting of build-ing up (creating new body tissue from food) and breaking down (deriving energy and creating waste products from tissue).

migraine (headache): A severe, throbbing headache, often recurring, that begins with spasm or constriction of the arteries in the skull. Migraine headaches are often accompanied by nausea and vomiting and sensitivity to light and sound.

morbidity (rate): The frequency or proportion of people with a particular diagnosis or disability in a given population.

myalgia: Pain of the muscles.

myofascial pain syndrome: Describes a localized area of muscle and surrounding tissue pain or tenderness.

narcotic: A class of drugs that reduce pain by blocking pain signals traveling from the central nervous system to the brain. While narcotics have the potential to be addictive and are abused by some people, they can be used safely for effective pain relief under skilled medical supervision.

neural hormones: Hormones produced in the brain and central nervous system. See also *hormones*.

nocturnal myoclonus: A benign type of seizure activity that usually occurs as a sudden jerk or thrash of the leg in the period of transition to sleep. These spasms happen to many people in the general population as well as in people with fibromyalgia, and they may disrupt sleep.

nonrestorative sleep: See *stages of sleep*.

NSAID (nonsteroidal anti-inflammatory drug): A type of drug that does not contain steroids but is used to relieve pain by reducing inflammation.

objective: Capable of being observed or measured; for example, infection can be objectively observed by the presence of bacteria in a blood test or culture test. See also *subjective*.

obstructive sleep apnea: See *sleep apnea*.

osteoarthritis: A disease causing cartilage breakdown in certain joints (spine, hands, hips, knees) resulting in pain and deformity.

pacing: Scheduling your daily tasks so that heavy and light tasks are alternated and work is balanced with rest.

pain: A sensation or perception of hurting, ranging from discomfort to agony, that occurs in response to injury, disease, or functional disorder. Pain is your body's alarm system, signaling that something is wrong. *Acute* pain is temporary and related to nerve endings stimulated by tissue damage and improves with healing. *Chronic* pain may be mild to severe but persists due to prolonged tissue damage or due to pain impulses that keep the pain gate open.

pediatrician: A physician with special training who specializes in the diagnosis, treatment and prevention of childhood and adolescent illness.

pediatric rheumatologist: See *rheumatologist*.

peptic ulcer: A benign (not cancerous) lesion in the stomach or duodenum that may cause pain, nausea, vomiting or bleeding. Such lesions can be caused by nonsteroidal anti-inflammatory drugs such as aspirin or ibuprofen.

perceived exertion: An individual's subjective measure of how much effort is required to perform a task.

physiatrist: A physician who specializes in the field of physical medicine and rehabilitation.

physical therapist: A person who has professional training and is licensed in the practice of physical therapy.

physical therapy: Methods and techniques of rehabilitation to restore function and prevent disability following injury or disease. Methods may include applications of heat and cold, assistive devices, massage and an individually tailored program of exercises.

pituitary: A small gland located at the base of the brain that secretes pituitary hormones. These hormones play a vital role in growth and development, in how the body stores and uses energy, and in the activity of other glands. See also *hormones.*

podiatrist: A health professional who specializes in care of the foot. Formerly called a chiropodist.

prioritizing: Choosing the most important activities or responsibilities; placing tasks in order so that your attention goes first to those that are most important or pressing.

progressive relaxation: A method of relieving muscle tension by focusing on one body part, then another, in sequence, usually beginning with the muscles of the toes and feet and ending with the facial muscles.

psychiatrist: A physician who trains after medical school in the study, treatment and prevention of mental disorders. A psychiatrist may provide counseling and prescribe medicines and other therapies.

psychologist: A trained professional, usually a PhD rather than an MD, who specializes in the mind and mental processes. A psychologist measures mental abilities and counsels, but may not prescribe drugs.

psychosomatic: Pertaining to the link between the mind (psyche) and the body (soma).

range of motion (ROM): The distance and angles at which your joints can be moved, extended, and rotated in various directions. Full or normal range of motion means that the joints move without impairment to their normal limits up, down, around, forward and back. Limited range of motion means that stiffness, pain or other problems interfere with free movement.

rapid eye movement (REM) sleep: The period of sleep in which people dream, occurring about every 90 minutes during normal sleep. It gets its name from rapid eye movements that occur under closed lids during this period. Scientists think that storage of information in long-term memory may also occur during REM sleep. See also *stages of sleep.*

Raynaud's phenomenon: Restriction of blood flow to the fingers, toes, or (rarely) to the nose or ears, in response to cold or emotional upset. This results in temporary blanching or paleness of the skin, tingling, numbness and pain.

reconditioning: Restoring or improving muscle tone and strength with appropriate and balanced exercise, nutrition, and rest. See also *deconditioning.*

relaxation: A state of release from mental or physical stress or tension.

REM: See *rapid eye movement (REM) sleep.*

remission: The term used to describe a period when symptoms of a disease or condition improve or even disappear.

repetitive strain injury: Pain caused by repeated muscle use.

restless legs syndrome: Peculiar crawling or spastic sensations in the legs that produce a need to move the legs; often worse in evenings.

rheumatic disease: A general term referring to conditions characterized by pain and stiffness of the joints or muscles. The American

College of Rheumatology currently recognizes over 100 rheumatic diseases.

rheumatoid arthritis: A chronic, inflammatory autoimmune disease in which the body's protective immune system turns on the body and attacks the joints, causing pain, swelling and deformity.

rheumatologist: A physician who pursues additional training after medical school and specializes in the diagnosis, treatment and prevention of arthritis and other rheumatic disorders. *Pediatric rheumatologist:* A rheumatologist who specializes in the diagnosis, treatment and prevention of arthritis or other rheumatic diseases in children and adolescents.

self-help: Any course, activity or action that you do for yourself to improve your circumstances or ability to cope with a situation.

self-talk: The voice in your head that you use to talk to yourself, out loud or in thought.

serotonin: A hormone that constricts blood vessels and contracts smooth muscle. See also *hormones, migraine (headache), SSRI, stages of sleep.*

skeletal muscles: The voluntary muscles that are primarily involved in moving parts of the body. "Voluntary" in this sense refers to muscles that move in response to our decisions to walk, bend, grasp and so on, as opposed to muscles such as the heart, which do their work without our willful direction.

sleep apnea: Cessation of breathing during sleep, caused by obstruction of the nasal airway, sometimes many times during the night. This condition is associated with obesity, but not all people who have sleep apnea are obese. Because the brain must arouse the sleeper from deep sleep to relieve the obstruction and restore breathing, sleep apnea has serious health effects.

social worker: A person who has professional training and is licensed to assist people in need by helping them capitalize on their own resources and connecting them with social services (for example, home nursing care or vocational rehabilitation).

soft-tissue rheumatism: Pertaining to the many rheumatic conditions affecting the soft (as opposed to the hard or bony) tissues of the body. Fibromyalgia is one type of soft-tissue rheumatism. Others are bursitis, tendinitis and focal myofascial pain.

somatomedin C (also called ICF-1): A hormone produced by the liver in response to growth hormone stimulation. Somatomedin C stimulates repair of muscle, bone and skin.

SSRI (selective serotonin reuptake inhibitor): A recently developed group of medications used to treat depression, including *Prozac* and *Zoloft*. These work by decreasing levels of serotonin in the brain and are sometimes better tolerated and perhaps more effective than other antidepressants.

stages of sleep: Four phases that occur and reoccur during a normal night of sleep, each characterized by specific types of brain wave activity. Stage 1 is a transition state between wakefulness and sleep. Stage 2 is the first level of true sleep. Stages 3 and 4 are the deepest, most restorative stages. Restorative sleep is sleep in which Stages 3 and 4 occur uninterrupted and promote renewal of health or sleep. Non-restorative sleep is sleep in which Stage 3 or 4 sleep is interrupted, shortened, or denied, thus denying the restorative benefits as well. See also *alpha wave, delta wave,* and *rapid eye movement (REM) sleep.*

steroids: A group name for lipids (fat substances) produced in the body and sharing a particular type of chemical structure. Among these are bile acids, cholesterol and some hormones. Not the same as anabolic steroids, drugs synthesized from testosterone (the male sex hormone), and used by some athletes to promote strength and endurance.

strain: Injury to a muscle, tendon or ligament by repetitive use, trauma, or excessive stretching.

strengthening exercises: Exercises that help maintain or increase muscle strength. See also *isometric exercises* and *isotonic exercises.*

stress: The result produced when the body is acted upon by excessive physical or emotional forces. The term is commonly used to denote either a cause or an effect.

subjective: Events or circumstances that are measured through one's personal perceptions but cannot be verified by objective measures. For example, pain in fibromyalgia can be felt and described but cannot be measured with a blood test, an X-ray or other tests. See also *objective.*

substance P: A molecule produced in the spinal cord in response to injury. Substance P stimulates nerve endings and produces pain, thus notifying the brain of injury and imminent danger.

sustained pain: See *pain.*

syndrome: A collection of symptoms and/or physical findings that characterize a particular abnormal condition or illness.

target heart rate: The number of heartbeats per minute that people want to reach during exercise in order to gain maximum benefits. Because the normal heart rate changes as we age, target heart rates are grouped by age.

tender-point injection: Injection of a painkilling medication directly into a tender point

BIBLIOGRAPHY

The following resources were used in preparation of this book.

Arthritis Foundation. *Fibromyalgia Self-Help Course*, class participant's manual. Atlanta, GA, 1995.

Arthritis Foundation. *Fibromyalgia Self-Help Course*, course leader's manual. Atlanta, GA, 1995.

Arthritis Foundation. *Primer on the Rheumatic Diseases.* 11th ed. Atlanta, GA, 1997.

Barsky, Arthur J., et al. "Functional Somatic Syndromes." *Annals of Internal Medicine*, 130 (11), June 1, 1999, pp. 910-921.

Bennett, Robert M. "Emerging Concepts in the Neurobiology of Chronic Pain: Evidence of Abnormal Sensory Processing in Fibromyalgia." *Mayo Clinical Procedures*, 74 (4), April 1999, pp. 385-98.

Bennett, Robert M. "The Fibromyalgia Syndrome: Myofascial Pain and the Chronic Fatigue Syndrome." In *Textbook of Rheumatology*, 4th ed., vol. 1, eds. W. N. Kelley, E. D. Harris Jr., S. Ruddy, and C. B. Sledge. Philadelphia, PA: W. B. Saunders Co., 1993, pp. 471-483.

Bennett, Robert M., Sharon R. Clark, Stephen M. Campbell, and Carol S.

Burckhardt. "Low Levels of Somatomedin C in Patients with the Fibromyalgia Syndrome." *Arthritis & Rheumatism*, Vol. 35, No. 10, Oct. 1992, p. 1113.

Bennett, Robert M., et. al. "A Randomized, Double-Blind, Placebo-Controlled Study of Growth Hormone in the Treatment of Fibromyalgia." *American Journal of Medicine,* 104 (3), March '98, pp. 227-31.

Berman, Brian M. et.al. "Is Acupuncture Effective in the Treatment of Fibromyalgia?" *Journal of Family Practice.* 48 (3), March 1999, pp. 213-218.

Bloomfield S. A., and E. F. Coyle. "Bed rest, detraining, and retention of training-induced adaptation." In ACSM's resource manual for guidelines for exercise testing and prescription, eds. J. L. Durstine, A. C. King, P. L. Painter, J. L. Roitman, and L. D. Zwiren. Philadelphia, PA: Lea and Febiger, 1993, pp. 115-128.

Boisset-Pioro, H. Mathilde, MD, CM; John M. Esdaile, MD, MPH; and Mary-Ann Fitzcharles, MD. "Sexual and Physical Abuse in Women with Fibromyalgia Syndrome." *Arthritis & Rheumatism*, Vol. 38, No. 2, Feb. 1995, pp. 235-241.

Buckelew SP, et. al. "Biofreedback/Relaxation Training and Exercise Interventions for Fibromyalgia: A Prospective Trial." *Arthritis Care*

Research. 11 (3), June 1998, pp. 196-209.

Burns, David, MD. *Feeling Good: The New Mood Therapy.* A Signet Book, 1980.

Buskila, Dan, et al. "Increased Rates of Fibromyalgia Following Cervical Spine Injury. *Arthritis & Rheumatism*, Vol 40, 3, March '97, pp. 446-452.

Carette, Simon. "Chronic Pain Syndromes." *Annals of the Rheumatic Diseases*, Vol. 55, 1996, pp. 497-501.

Covertino, VA, et. al. "An Overview of the Issues: Physiological Effects of Bed Rest and Restricted Physical Activity." *Medical Science and Sports Exercise.* 29 (2), Feb. 1997, pp 187-190.

Crofford, Leslie J. "Neuroendocrine Abnormalities in Fibromyalgia and Related Disorders." *American Journal of Medical Science,* 315 (6), June 1998, pp. 359-66.

Dorland's Illustrated Medical Dictionary. 28th ed. Philadelphia, PA: W. B. Saunders Co., 1994.

Dunkin, Mary Anne. "Fibromyalgia Comes Out of the Closet." *Arthritis Today*, Sept.-Oct. 1993, pp. 24-28.

Dunkin, Mary Anne, ed. "New Clues to the Cause of Fibromyalgia." *Arthritis Today.* Mar.-Apr. 1993, p. 10.

Educational Rights for Children with Arthritis-Related Conditions publication. Atlanta, GA:

Arthritis Foundation, 1996. Foltz-Gray, Dorothy. "Comic Relief." *Arthritis Today.* Nov.-Dec. 1998, pp.26-30.

Fransen, RN, Jenny, and I. Jon Russell, MD. *The Fibromyalgia Help Book: Practical Guide to Living Better with Fibromyalgia.* St. Paul, MN: Smith House Press, 1996.

Goldenberg, Don, et. al. "A Randomized, Double-Blind Crossover Trial of Fluoxetine and Amitriptyline in the Treatment of Fibromyalgia." *Arthritis & Rheumatism.* Vol 39 (11), Nov. 1996, pp. 1852-1859.

Gowens, SE et. al. "A Randomized, Controlled Trial of Exercise and Eduction for Individuals with Fibromyalgia." *Arthritis Care Research.* 12 (2), April 1999, pp. 120-128.

Grady, Eugene P. "Rheumatic Finding in Gulf War Veterans." *Archives of Internal Medicine.* 158 (4), Feb. 23, '98, pp. 367-7l.

Hench, MD, P. Kahler. "Sleep and Rheumatic Disease." *Bulletin on the Rheumatic Diseases,* Vol. 45, No. 8, Dec. 1996. pp. 1-5.

Hudson, James I., MD, and Harrison G. Pope Jr., MD. "Does Childhood Sexual Abuse Cause Fibromyalgia?" *Arthritis & Rheumatism,* Vol. 38, No. 2, Feb. 1995, pp. 161-163.

Kelley, W. N., Ed Harris Jr., S. Ruddy, and C. B. Sledge, eds. *Textbook of Rheumatology.* 5th ed.

Philadelphia, PA: W. B. Saunders Co., 1997. Kübler-Ross, E. *On Death and Dying*. New York: Macmillan Publishing Co., 1981. Mikkelsson, Marja. "One Year Outcome of Preadolescents with Fibromyalgia." *The Journal of Rheumatology,* 26:3, pp. 674-682.

National Arthritis Data Workgroup, unpublished data, 1997.

Pennebaker, MD, James W. *Opening Up: The Healing Power of Confiding in Others.* New York: Avon Books, 1990.

Physician's Desk Reference. 50th ed. Montvale, NJ: Medical Economics Co., 1996.

Potera, Carol. "Fibromyalgia Finding." *Arthritis Today*, Jan.-Feb. 1995, p. 9.

Russell, I. J., J. E. Michalek, G. A. Vipraio, E. M. Fletcher, M. A. Javors, and C. A. Bowden. "Platelet 3H-Imipramine Uptake Receptor Density and Serum Serotonin Levels in Patients with Fibromyalgia/ Fibrositis Syndrome." *Journal of Rheumatology*. Vol. 19, 1992, pp. 104-109.

Russell I. J., H. Vaeroy, M. Javors, and F. Nyberg. "Cerebrospinal Fluid Biogenic Amine Metabolites in Fibromyalgia/Fibrositis Syndrome and Rheumatoid Arthritis." *Arthritis & Rheumatism,* Vol. 35, 1992, pp. 550-556.

Russell I. J., G. A. Vipraio, E. M. Fletcher, Y. M. Lopez, M. D. Orr, and J. E. Michalek. "Characteristics of Spinal Fluid, Substance P

and Calcitonin Gene Related Peptide in Fibromyalgia Syndrome." *Arthritis & Rheumatism.* Vol. 39(9supp): Abstract 1485. Sherry, David D. "Pain Syndromes." *Adolescent Rheumatology.* pp. 197-217.

Simms, MD, Robert W. "Fibromyalgia Syndrome: Current Concepts in Pathophysiology, Clinical Features, and Management." *Arthritis Care and Research,* Vol. 9, No.4, Aug. 1996, pp. 315-328.

Simms, MD, Robert W., et. al. "Lack of Association Between Fibromyalgia Syndrome and Abnormalities in Muscle Enerby Metabolism." *Arthritis & Rheumatism*, Vol. 37, 6, June 1994, pp. 794-800.

Stedman's Medical Dictionary, 25th Ed., Illustrated. Baltimore, MD: Williams & Wilkins, 1990.

Taylor, Mary Lou, PhD, Dana R. Trotter, MD, and M. E. Csuka, MD. "The Prevalence of Sexual Abuse in Women with Fibromyalgia." *Arthritis & Rheumatism*, Vol. 38, No. 2, Feb. 1995, pp. 229-234. *Textbook of Rheumatology.* 3rd ed. Philadelphia, PA: W. B. Saunders Co., 1990.

Wolfe, Frederick, Kathryn Ross, Janice Anderson, I. Jon Russell, and Liesi Hebert. "The Prevalence and Characteristics of Fibromyalgia in the General Population." *Arthritis & Rheumatism*, Vol. 38, No. 1, Jan. 1995, pp. 19-28.

Yunus, M.B. "Genetic Factors in Fibromyalgia Syndrome." *The Journal of Rheumatology.* 26. 1999, pp. 408-412.

Yunus, M. B., and A. T. Masic. "Juvenile Primary Fibromyalgia Syndrome: A Clinical Study of Thirty-Three Patients and Matched Normal Controls." *Arthritis & Rheumatism,* Vol. 28, 1985, pp. 138-145.

INDEX

RESOURCES FOR GOOD LIVING

The mission of the Arthritis Foundation is to improve lives through leadership in the prevention, control and cure of arthritis and related diseases.

As a nonprofit organization, the Arthritis Foundation relies on your contributions to fund research, programs and services. You can make a difference in people's lives by becoming a member of the Arthritis Foundation. Please contact your local chapter or call 800/933-0032. You will receive materials about the benefits of Arthritis Foundation membership, including the award-winning bimonthly magazine Arthritis Today. Log on to the Foundation Web site, www.arthritis.org, for more information about arthritis, Arthritis Foundation resources or to find the chapter nearest you.

Programs and Services

Physician referral - Most Arthritis Foundation chapters can provide a list of doctors in your area who specialize in the evaluation and treatment of arthritis and arthritis-related diseases.

Exercise programs - The Arthritis Foundation sponsors, develops and coordinates exercise programs for people with arthritis, featuring specially trained instructors. These programs include:

- Walk With Ease - This course, accompanied by a book, shows you ways to develop a walking routine for fitness.

- *PACE** (People with Arthritis Can Exercise)- These courses feature gentle movements to increase joint flexibility, range of motion, stamina and muscle strength. An accompanying video is available for home use.

- Arthritis Foundation Aquatic Program -These water exercise programs help relieve strain on muscles and joints. An accompanying PEP (Pool Exercise Program) video is available for home use.

Educational and Support Groups - The Arthritis Foundation sponsors mutual-support groups that provide opportunities for discussion and problem-

solving among people with arthritis. In addition, the Arthritis Foundation offers courses designed to help people actively manage their particular disease through exercise, medications, relaxation techniques, pain management, nutrition and more. These classes include the Arthritis Self-Help Course and the Fibromyalgia Self-Help Course.

Information and Products

Find the latest information about arthritis, including research, medications, government advocacy, programs and services, through one of the many information resources offered by the Arthritis Foundation:

www.arthritis.org

Information about arthritis is available 24 hours a day on the Internet at the Arthritis Foundation's interactive, comprehensive Web site. Find news about arthritis, ways to get involved, and a variety of useful arthritis products, including books, brochures, videos and more. In addition, the Arthritis Foundation has a new interactive self-management guide for people with arthritis, Connect and Control: Your Online Arthritis Action Guide. Via questionnaire responses, Connect and Control helps participants create a customized management program for their unique challenges. Participants may use Connect and Control to create their own customized health-assessment program.

Arthritis Answers

Call toll-free at 800/283-7800 for 24-hour, automated information about arthritis and Arthritis Foundation resources. Trained volunteers and staff also are available at your local Arthritis Foundation chapter to answer questions or refer you to physicians and other resources. For general questions about arthritis, you also can call 404/872-7100, Ext. 1, or email questions to help@arthritis.org.

Publications

The Arthritis Foundation offers many publications to educate people with arthritis, as well as their families and friends, about diagnosis, medications, exercise, diet, pain management and more.

- Books - The Arthritis Foundation publishes a variety of books on arthritis to help you understand and manage your condition, live a healthier life, and cope with the emotional challenges that come with a chronic illness. Order books directly at www.arthritis.org, or by calling 800/207-8633. All Arthritis Foundation books are available in retail bookstores.

- Brochures - The Arthritis Foundation offers brochures containing concise, understandable information on the many arthritis-related diseases and conditions. Topics include surgery, the latest medications, guidance for working with your doctors, and self-managing your illness. Single copies are available free of charge at www.arthritis.org, or by calling 800/283-7800.

- Arthritis Today - This award-winning, bimonthly magazine provides interesting feature articles in each issue, providing the latest information on research, new treatments, trends and tips from experts and readers to help you manage arthritis. A one-year subscription to Arthritis Today is included as a benefit when you become a member of the Arthritis Foundation. Annual membership is $25 and helps fund research to find cures for arthritis. Call 800/933-0032 for information.

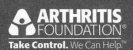